What Readers are Saying

"When my young husband of eight months died by suicide, I searched for a resource to help me to cope. I scanned bookstores for weeks and left empty-handed. In 1987, no one talked about suicide and no one wrote about surviving such a loss. I remember feeling confused and alone. The worst part was that I also felt ashamed. Then, I struggled with being ashamed of being ashamed. (He was dead, I thought, and here I was, selfishly feeling ashamed.)

Michelle's books are exactly what I needed at that time. And, they are exactly what our world needs right now! Expertly-written, these books are filled with important information and practical strategies for both the surviving spouse or partner and for those who are supporting a surviving spouse or partner."

Deri Latimer, B.Mgt.(HR), CSP
Spouse Suicide Loss Survivor
Author of *Not Crazy, Just Human:*
Moving Through Trauma to Healing

"This inspiring book shines a light into the darkness of grief from suicide loss. Michelle uses the tools of her professional coaching practice, along with her personal story of loss, to guide others on the path of healing."

Carole Marie Downing, MS, ND
Author of *Singing Beyond Sorrow,*
A Year of Grief, Gratitude & Grace

"Michelle shows us how she transformed her life after her loss in this thoughtful, inspiring, and deeply personal book. Her stories highlight how healing is possible."

Kristin A. Meekhof, LCSW
Coauthor of *A Widow's Guide to Healing:*
Gentle Support and Advice for the First 5 Years

"In *Surviving Spouse or Partner Suicide Loss,* Michelle shares her personal heart-wrenching experience of losing her husband to suicide and the journey she undertook to climb out from under the landslide of emotions and trauma left in the aftermath. Michelle bravely and tenderly conveys all this while empowering the reader with an incredible number of tools and techniques for embarking on their own journey of survival and healing."

Lori Giesey
Author of *A Moment In Time*

Surviving Spouse or Partner Suicide Loss

A Mindful Guide for Your Journey through Grief

Michelle Ann Collins

Saved By Story

Surviving Spouse or Partner Suicide Loss
A Mindful Guide for Your Journey through Grief

Published by
Saved By Story Publishing, LLC
Prescott, AZ

www.SavedByStory.house

Copyright © 2022 by Michelle Ann Collins

Cover by Alyssa Noelle Coelho
Interior Design by Dawn Teagarden
Photo by Jennifer Alyse

ISBN
Paperback: 979-8-9869578-3-8
eBook: 979-8-9869578-4-5

Printed in the United States of America
www.SavedByStory.house

This book is dedicated to you, the reader, for making the most difficult choice to journey toward healing. Your strength is inspiring. You are a true survivor.

Acknowledgments

Gratitude creates the threads from which we weave the tapestry of a joyful life.

I am grateful to you for holding this book in your hand; may it offer you some comfort on your journey.

I am grateful to everyone with whom I have shared mine. Whether a helper or an obstacle, you are my teacher, and you have contributed to my resilience and strength.

I am grateful to Amanda Johnson and the book doulas at True to Intention and Saved By Story Publishing. Without your help, this book would have been stuck in labor forever.

Gratitude also to three of my greatest teachers and mentors, David Kessler, Kristin Meehkof, and Linda Z. Your guidance has lightened my burdens so I could continue to heal. Your ability to shine a flashlight into the pitch blackness of my grief cave and others walking a similar path will inspire me always.

Contents

Part 3 | The Climb

INTRODUCTIONS

Crawling into the Cave

The Grief Cave

Allow me to send you a big virtual hug. I am truly sorry this book has come into your world because it means you have suffered a terrible loss. I am happy, however, that you have found it because it will help you realize you are not alone on this painful journey. It is meant to help ease your suffering and support you on your path toward healing.

My husband, Glen Collins, died by suicide in 2016. Recovering from the grief and trauma of this loss sent my life in a completely new and frightening direction. In this book, I share the knowledge and skills I gained during my journey. My goal is to help other suicide loss survivors have a more educated and, therefore, easier journey. When discussing my partner, I use he or him because I lost my husband; when addressing your partner or others, I use they or them. Please feel free to mentally change the pronoun and relationship details to suit your specific situation.

Context is required for understanding. At first, I had absolutely no context for this experience. As a writer and teacher, I often use metaphors to simplify complex concepts and "wrap my head around" difficult pieces of information or challenging experiences. I've come to think of the weeks, months, and years after Glen's death as picking myself up from a shocking fall. It was as if the ground beneath me had just disappeared and I had fallen into a dark, scary, lonely place. At first, I couldn't even grasp where I was or how I got there because the darkness was so thick and all-consuming.

Have you experienced days, weeks, months, or maybe even years during which you can't get your brain to even understand what happened?

**That's what I'm talking about.
I call that place the grief cave.**

After Glen's death, I tried to figure out how to stitch my body, mind, and soul back together. I had to do it mostly on my own, save for a few helpers. One of the most difficult things about the grieving process is that no one truly knows what you're going through. Even though your helpers may have experienced grief and loss, this loss is uniquely yours. Plus, many of them are dealing with the shock of their own fall *and* a gross lack of education about how to help someone through the experience of trauma and grief. Understandably you may feel isolated, but you are not alone. It *is* possible to get the support you need. You're already doing it by reading this.

I'll help you find your way out of the darkness. You are not alone.

In the beginning, I was buried by grief, trauma, and sorrow in my grief cave, and I rejected the whole idea of a new life. I thought I would never want to see the sky or feel the warmth of life again. My supporters (friends and therapists) pointed me toward the supplies, skills, and tools I needed to begin my journey out of the darkness, but starting the journey had to come from me. The shift toward healing happened when I realized I was obligated to continue on to live a full life. I needed to continue on because I still have a life to live. And to truly honor Glen's memory, I need to live the best life I can.

In this book, I share the knowledge I gained on my journey to healing as well as practices I used and continue using to help

me live a fulfilling life every day. I still experience grief, but there is also love and joy. World-renowned grief expert David Kessler reminds us that to live fully, we must grieve fully. I pray the tools that helped me process the trauma and pain and helped me grow strong enough to emerge from the cave and journey forward on a healing path can now support you as well.

We'll start in the grief cave—that dark, lonely place that feels so isolated and hopeless—and I will show you the supplies you need to use to move out of the cave. When you leave the cave and begin the next leg of your journey of healing, it will be beneficial to have a set of practices that will help you rest, assess, and release burdens when the journey and that grief backpack you are carrying is burdensome. Then you will begin the climb up some of the most important hidden staircases in the grief process. Climbing comes with pitfalls, switchbacks, obstacles, and unexpected interference. A byproduct of climbing, however, is gaining insight and strength into the climb itself, so when you meet obstacles, you can maneuver around them or find someone or something that can help remove them or make them manageable. Finally, you will summit. You will reach that place where the love outweighs the pain. From this beautiful place, where your heart and life are full, you will hold your loss close to you and honor it—and your strength—with love and grace.

Honoring Your Cave

I don't know that a book like this would have helped me in the earliest days after Glen's death—the "acute" phase of grief. I probably would have thrown it across the room in disbelief that some well-meaning friend was brazen enough to give me a how-to-get-through-it book when I believed there was no *through*.

I believed I would always feel as awful as I did on that terrible day Glen died. My world turned completely upside down, and I felt nothing but pain. I believed I was the only person who had ever felt such pain. "How could a total stranger know anything about how I'm feeling or what I need?" would have been my likely response. I wouldn't have believed anything could help. I imagine, from the depths of darkness I was inhabiting, I would have said something like "What am I supposed to do with this? I can't read a book and think about healing. I don't even know how to get out of bed and put on my shoes right now!"

As time went on, and there's no telling when this might happen for you, I realized I wanted to feel better—I *needed* to feel better. I understood that I was still alive and had an obligation to continue living *my* life. I knew I didn't want to stay in the grief cave forever. And I needed a guide to help me find my way out.

I had friends helping me with various tasks—first, the tasks of daily living, like eating and driving, and then helping me get out of the house to remember there was life outside. Then I had attorneys, accountants, and financial advisors helping me with the estate legalities, as well as clerks at the various government agencies, banks, and medical facilities where I needed to clear estate paperwork. I also had a great trauma therapist and a kind and caring coach.

What I didn't have was the warm support of someone who had been through it—someone to hold the flashlight for me and show me the path out of the darkness.

I promise you there is a path, and when you are ready, you will find it. This book and the stories and practices I share can be that guide for you.

A Guide with a Flashlight and More

When my mother died in 2007 after suffering from leukemia, I was sure that was the worst thing that would ever happen to me. After her diagnosis in 2003, I felt like the light went out of my life, and throughout her treatment, it rarely returned. I felt so lost and was suffering more deeply than I thought possible. My yoga practice was my refuge. After her death, I sought out deeper learning in yoga and started teaching in 2008. The more yoga I practiced and learned and taught, the more ease and fulfillment I brought into my life.

Meditation and mindfulness, especially breath awareness, are part of a well-rounded yoga practice. These practices sustained me through tough times, my divorce, my marriage to Glen, and painful estrangements that some of my relationships suffered.

Losing Glen caused an unimaginable amount of suffering. Between the trauma of our struggles leading up to his death, discovering his body, the complexities of his estate, and trying to help his family, my family, our friends, I got completely overwhelmed. To ease my suffering, I turned to substances and irresponsible behaviors. As you can imagine, this only impeded my progress toward healing. Finally, when I landed in my trauma therapist's office after a devastating threat by a friend to put me into rehab, I realized I was on the wrong path—one that led to self-destruction, not healing. Even though healing seemed like

an impossibility at the time, I knew my therapist was a signpost pointing in the right direction. And because my deepest desire was to feel better, I followed her advice. With her unfailing support and yoga, meditation, and mindfulness practices, I quit abusing substances and set out to find as many tools as I could that would ease my suffering and promote my healing journey.

In March 2017, I attended a retreat at The Chopra Center for Wellbeing called "A Journey into Healing." Afterward, I began to feel deep and profound changes. It took time and commitment, but as I said, I was going to try anything (legal and healthy this time) to feel better. The retreat helped me more fully understand the connection between experience, processing experience, and health and disease. I began to see my body as one part of a much bigger whole. I realized that the emotional trauma I experienced was living in my body and, if not processed and healed, the grief and trauma I was experiencing—my dis-ease—would likely become disabling physical and mental disease.

I started studying meditation more deeply and expanded my studies into spirituality and consciousness. I'll share more about the specifics throughout the book, but my main point here is that in order to feel good again (yes, it's possible) and to heal (absolutely possible), I had to make a real effort to understand what happened to me when I experienced trauma. I had to realize that the experience of losing Glen deeply affected not only my emotional well-being but my physical, mental, and spiritual well-being as well.

I went on to study Ayurveda at the Chopra Center and got a certification in Ayurvedic lifestyle education. I studied yoga for trauma as well as the neuroscience of trauma and grief, and in order to have more tools and learn the language of grief so I could help others, I became a certified grief educator. Working as

a grief and wellness coach, I continue to increase my knowledge of and dedication to healing trauma and grief.

I know it may not seem believable right now, but healing *is* possible! Healing doesn't mean forgetting your loved one or moving away from them or your love for them. It only means you can live a fulfilling and joyful life with their memory—the new form of your relationship with them.

> **Helpful Tip:** Just because your loved one died doesn't mean your relationship with them is over. It is changed forever, as are you, but you can still hold them close in your heart. Many people who lose their partner or spouse say they are still married, and their spouse is in heaven. You can try this out and see how it feels. This idea may seem ridiculous, or it may feel right on. Try it on and see if it feels right to you.

I'm including mindfulness tools, other health-related insights, and grief support in this book because, frankly, I don't know any other way to navigate healing.

If any of the tools in this book don't seem useful or seem too much to you, just skip them for now. You can come back to them later. When you are ready, they'll be here. Meanwhile, take care of yourself the best you can.

The Truth about Grief and Trauma

There are differences between trauma and grief that, if understood, can give you insight into your experience. While we grieve most losses, especially the loss of a loved one to death, we don't always experience trauma with the loss of a loved one.

Grief is hard. We feel a loss, and it can send us into deep sadness. We ache for our loved one, and even though we know they will not return, we yearn for their company. It takes a long time for our minds to fully understand our loss. Grief can be filled with so many emotions: sadness, guilt, regret, even love and joy from a happy memory. Grievers may experience anxiety, brain fog, difficulty recalling things, or disorientation. All these are perfectly normal and will take time to resolve. If you find you still have an inability to do normal daily tasks after some time (months, years—it's different for everyone), professional help in the form of a grief therapist, counselor, or coach is a good idea.

Grief is not a disease; it's a natural process we go through when we experience loss. You are not sick; you are in grief.

Because suicide loss survivors almost always experience trauma, it is helpful to understand what happens in our bodies and minds when we are challenged by a traumatic experience. When we are traumatized, our nervous system gets overwhelmed and goes into

a mode that tries to protect us from further damage. Think of it like a circuit breaker. Have you ever had too many things plugged in and running at once and the power to the whole circuit went out? Everything stops, and you have to unplug the items that caused the overload and reset the circuit breaker. This is where most of us are after the trauma of suicide loss. A trauma like this in adulthood can also activate* us to remember or feel traumatic childhood experiences or even unresolved compound losses from our adulthood.

> ***Language is important and impactful.** The words we use and hear can have a strong effect on how we feel. As the suicide awareness community shifts from using the term "committed suicide" to "died by suicide," there has also been a shift in the trauma community around the word "trigger." I personally really appreciate this shift because, since Glen died by using a gun, even the word "trigger" used to activate my trauma response. Talk about adding pain to pain. Now the trauma world is shifting to using the word "activated." I'm so grateful for this shift. Think about the word. If something gets activated, you get into your fight-or-flight response, but there are ways, as I'll discuss in detail in this book, to deactivate it. Once a trigger is pulled, there's no taking it back. I'm working on making this shift myself. Try it on and see how "activated" feels. If you're like me, you will feel better using it. I feel it is much softer and promotes healing.

In addition to recovering from trauma, the complex grief that can be uniquely a part of suicide loss makes healing that much more challenging. When my mother died from leukemia, I felt many

of the things one would expect after a loss. Guilt: "I could have taken better care of her while she was suffering." Sadness: "I miss her so much." Hopelessness: "I will never be happy again," and "I can't live without her." Grieving future losses: "She won't see my kids graduate or get married or meet her great-grandchildren." But never did I think, "Oh, if only I hadn't _____, she wouldn't have gotten cancer." or "If I had just driven her to the doctor one more time, she wouldn't have died." Part of the challenge of any loss is guilt, but when we look at suicide, our mind can trick us into believing we could have had a greater effect on the outcome. Suicide loss is accompanied by extreme guilt because of the mistaken belief that we could have prevented the suicide from happening. *We would have prevented it if we could have.* Grief expert David Kessler says, "We would rather be guilty than helpless."[1]

We are helpless to stop our spouse's suicide, but we are *not* guilty of causing it. The cause of suicide is most often mental illness, and our spouse/partner's mental illness is never our fault.

It is not because we didn't pick up the phone that one time. It is not because we left them alone or lived separately or messed up their dinner order.

There is nothing we could have done differently. Another hospitalization, another physician, another medication, another vacation, another conversation—all these things might have helped, or they might not have. The truth is that if someone is determined to die, they will, and we cannot stop it.

We cannot change the fact that our loved one has died. There is, however, a big something we *do* have control over. We can figure out how to go on from here—to heal, to grow our hearts and minds and lives around the loss, and to find meaning in our lives to honor our lost loved ones.

Here's a bit of neurobiology to help explain what is happening in your mind and body:

The part of the nervous system that controls our breathing, heartbeat, digestion, and perspiration, among other things, is called our autonomic nervous system. When we are faced with a challenge, our autonomic nervous system responds by kicking many systems into high gear. Tasked with keeping us alive, it responds as if we're being chased by a bear and running for, or about to fight for, our lives. Our heart rate increases; breathing becomes more like hyperventilating, preparing our muscles for battle; blood clots faster (in case of an attack to keep us from bleeding to death); and digestion shuts down (we don't need to process our most recent meal when we're running for our lives). It's the same with our immune system and our higher functioning brain. We don't need to fight off a cold or do geometry or reason through complicated problems when we are either going to be lunch, fighting not to be lunch, or running to hide behind a tree to escape from being lunch.

That's the beauty and the curse of our nervous system's preprogrammed response to stress. Our stress response increases our chances of survival when our lives are under immediate threat. The problem, however, is this response was meant to last only a few minutes, not weeks, months, or even years. When we cannot manage stress and regulate our nervous system, we experience chronic dis-ease. We get sick. Our complex and powerful stress response evolved to work very short-term to save our lives. But when it lasts beyond a few minutes, it can make us barely able to think or make decisions, anxious, depressed, or even unaware of our current surroundings.

Right now (and maybe for months before your partner died, if things were rocky), you may be deep in trauma, shock, and grief.

Have you noticed, in the stress of grief, how difficult it is to do what used to be really simple tasks? How about getting good sleep? While you're being chased by a bear? Not likely. It's because your body is putting all its resources into preparing for fight or flight, not reasoning how to make a spreadsheet of the estate bills, planning anything, or relaxing enough to go into rest-and-digest mode.

The definition of trauma is that your nervous system has been overwhelmed by your experience, and this can lead to dissociation. Dissociation is a trauma response where you separate mentally and emotionally from your current situation because your nervous system is overwhelmed and cannot take any further input. This can show up as anything from being distracted and unable to concentrate, to memory issues, to full-blown flashbacks where you revisit the traumatic event and it feels like you are actually there. It can be very upsetting.

The tools included in this book will help settle your nervous system so the natural process of grief can unfold.

The Purpose of This Survival Guide

Sadly, suicide is becoming more and more common. With the increases in suicide loss and suicide loss awareness, communities have sprouted on social media. I'm so glad to see more and more places to find global community support for suicide loss. When I lost Glen, I felt completely isolated in my grief. I didn't know how to grieve, and I didn't have a grieving community. And when I reached out to my usual supporters—friends, families, yoga family, and synagogue—all the support I got was intermingled with my supporters' feelings about Glen and his death. No one could figure out or tell me how to move forward, what direction to go, and how to get there to begin healing.

To support your survival and eventual healing, this guide puts all the tools I have learned and used into a single resource for you. One of the most important things I want to share is that no two grief experiences are the same. That includes my experience, your experience, and the experience of anyone else who may also be grieving the loss of your spouse or partner. A tool that might help them may not help you. Keep seeking until you find a set of tools that helps you feel like you're on the path to healing. Believe you will find them. You're already here reading this, so you are well on your way.

Permission Slips

In *Dare to Lead*, Brené Brown eloquently describes permission slips, and they are a valuable tool we can use on our journey.[2] Early on, I realized I needed to give myself some grief-focused permission slips to move through this process. Here are a few to consider, but feel free to write ones that resonate with you:

Slip 1: It's okay to be where I am.

If you can give yourself permission to be where you are, it will help lessen your suffering. How do you know where you are? Imagine arriving at a brand-new grocery store. You typically need a moment to orient yourself to where the produce, dairy, and other food aisles are so you can find everything on your grocery list.

When we are thrust into the trauma of suicide loss, we are unprepared. The grief and shock are overwhelming, and with the trauma connected to suicide and spouse/partner loss on top of it—of course you're lost! But you are lost *somewhere*. And figuring that out first and foremost will help you identify the kind of help you need to begin the next phase of your life with as much ease and hope for healing as possible. If you take time to assess your situation, you will feel more in control.

To get an idea of where you are, try answering the following questions regarding the immediate moment:

Yes   No   I have a place to live.

Yes   No   I have food for my next meal.

Yes   No   My immediate family and I are safe.

Yes   No   I am breathing. (I wanted you
             to have an easy one.)

Yes   No   I have someone I can hug during
             the next twenty-four hours.

Slip 2: I give myself permission to feel all the feelings. No feelings are wrong; they are simply how I feel.

I like to think of emotions as energy in motion. Check in with yourself right now. I bet you don't feel exactly the same as you did this morning, or yesterday, or a month ago. Feelings, emotions, come and go. This fact has helped get me through the most difficult times. I say to myself, *I will not always feel the way I feel now.* At times, that is the only help I could be to myself.

Perhaps you had no idea the suicide was coming and are completely shocked. Your partner may have threatened suicide, but you never believed they would go through with it. You may be so deep in sadness that you can't feel anything else. Are you angry? Are you afraid? It may have been a terrifying time. You may have complicated and confusing feelings. Possibly along with grief and loss and trauma, you could feel some relief—for the end of your partner's suffering or perhaps for the end of the trauma you endured through abuse and threats to your safety.

You may be feeling all those feelings mixed in with heartbreaking guilt and shame. It's okay. None of those feelings are bad or wrong. They are simply how you feel.

And if you do not feel terrible right at this moment, that's okay too.

It is easy to confuse the meanings of shame and guilt and very important to understand the difference between them.

You are experiencing shame when you say something like, "I'm a terrible person for not answering the phone the last time they called."

Guilt would say something more like, "I feel terrible that I didn't answer the phone."

When we feel shame, we feel we are unworthy or a "bad" person.

When we feel guilt, we regret something we did and wish we could go back and change it. We may be mad at ourself or feel sad about our actions, but we don't feel that gut punch of unworthiness, fear, or isolation.

Any feelings you are feeling are okay!

If your loss happened in recent months, you're likely in survival mode, even if you don't recognize it as such due to the foggy brain state that survival mode can create. You may feel lost as far as knowing what to do or what steps to take to begin to find any feelings of normalcy or hope in this jarring new phase of your life. You may be experiencing what feels like a fog that shrouds much of what's going on. It's okay; the fog will lift when it's time. But right now, this fog is protecting you. It's your brain's

way of filtering and keeping you from overwhelm—keeping those parts that overloaded the system unplugged from the circuit. It's saying, "Hey, I can't handle any more right now, so I'm going to let only the basics through. Everything else can wait until I've had some time to process, integrate, and get stronger." Resisting this fog or trying to force it to go away is usually an exercise in futility, leading us to even less clarity and more stress. Allow yourself to be in this mode for as long as you need. Think of it as a protective, healing cocoon. Take care of the basics, which I'll list in the coming pages, and let go of everything you possibly can. The details, challenges, and tasks will be there waiting for you when the fog clears and you develop the strength you need to tackle them. It *will* get easier!

> **Don't beat yourself up because you aren't feeling the way you or the people around you are expecting you to feel. (Talk about adding insult to injury.)**

So many times during these last few years, I felt I was alone in my grief and that I just couldn't go on. I knew hardly anyone my age (I was fifty at the time of Glen's death) who had lost a spouse, much less to suicide. Further isolating was the fact he was my second husband (we'd been married less than two years), and due to difficult circumstances in our relationship, we were living separately when he died. Glen and I had fallen in love so quickly and so intensely, only a year after my divorce, that we rushed into marriage ninety days after we met. This destabilized or destroyed almost every remaining post-divorce relationship I had, leading to estrangements from my family, friends, and community. When he died such a short time later, I was even more isolated because of these estrangements. This intensified my feelings of guilt and shame to the point that I wondered if I even deserved to grieve. On top of the trauma of losing him this way and the grief, I berated

myself and dragged myself deeper and deeper into the perilous shadow of shame and guilt. And I wish I hadn't.

Let me reassure you that *any* feelings you are having are completely okay. *You have every right to grieve*, however you need to, regardless of the circumstances before your partner's death. No one can tell you what is right or wrong about your grieving, how long to grieve, or how to move forward with your life. Don't believe for a second you are not entitled to any feelings you are having. Mental/emotional pain is just as legitimate as physical pain; in fact, you may be feeling physical pain because of your shock and grief. You are injured. If you had broken your leg, would you continually beat the broken leg with a stick? Would you tell your leg it's really dumb for breaking? No, you would nurture your leg and let it heal so you can get back to walking and all the great stuff you miss doing because your leg is broken. Grief is like that: If you nurture yourself and take care of your mind, emotions, and body, your healing will thrive.

The best thing you can do right now is care for yourself, not beat yourself up with guilt, shame, or other self-harming emotions. Take care of yourself so you can heal.

To help yourself, focus on finding a way to ease your suffering and begin your recovery. Slow down. You don't have to do everything at once. Treat your mind and body gently! When the fog clears enough for you to want to search for the next step, the guidance offered in this book will help you find some direction and comfort.

Checking in with how you are feeling is also part of the assessment that will help you on your journey. Feelings, although they can be really intense, are always temporary. They come and go. I promise, you will not always feel the way you feel right now. Keeping in mind that every feeling you're experiencing is

completely legitimate, use the following questions to get an idea of how you feel at this moment:

Yes   No   I feel angry.

Yes   No   I feel afraid.

Yes   No   I feel sad.

Yes   No   I feel heavy.

Yes   No   I feel relieved. (Yes, you have permission to feel even this.)

Yes   No   I feel upset.

Yes   No   I feel tired.

Yes   No   I feel calm.

Yes   No   I feel nothing.

Being aware of your feelings and naming them can actually lessen their intensity and allow you to feel a little more in control.

Slip 3: I give myself permission to move through my grieving journey in the way and at the pace that most supports my healing.

Spouse or partner loss, and especially suicide loss, is a unique and complex experience. You may feel many losses piled on top of each other. It's possible that you lost your greatest love, or the source of your fear, or your soulmate, or your greatest challenge. It could be a combination. With this single act, not only did your spouse or partner die, but your relationship status changed as well. This person was your primary relationship. This is a massive

shock, and it might take years to realize and accept. Do you despise the term "suicide widow"? It's okay to never identify as a widow, much less a suicide widow. The answer to this question may also change over time, and guess what? That's okay! Give yourself permission to find out who you are now and how to identify yourself, and do it in your own time.

Only you get to make these decisions; this next stage of your life is up to *you*. When you're ready, the following statements may help you discover your current identity and begin orienting you toward your new life. As you read them, see if they resonate. If they don't, that's okay too!

I am:

___ married, and my spouse/partner is in heaven.

___ a widow, and my husband died suddenly.

___ a widow, and my husband died by suicide.

___ single

___ not ready to decide what my current identity is.

_____(fill in your own).

Your answers may shift and change as you journey through grief. That's okay! Clarity will come, and when it does, relief will follow.

Slip 4: I give myself permission to consider that rebuilding is possible.

I know it's probably a weird time to think about this, but you *can* come through this situation with new self-awareness and health practices that create a stronger, more resilient you. Why

on earth would this be a time for self-improvement? Think of it as rebuilding your house after a fire. If everything had been destroyed, would you refill the house with the ugly old furniture and aged appliances that didn't bring you joy? If you had to rebuild, wouldn't you try to make the house as comfortable, functional, health-supporting, and beautiful as possible? It's your house, it's your life, and you can choose to use this as an opportunity to nurture your strengths and discard the parts of your life that sap your energy and don't support your health. You can build a sturdy, comfortable house using new tools that can ultimately make life easier to live and bring meaning to your experiences. But first, the basics: How do you get through this awful time?

It may sound impossible right now, but in time, you'll be able to accept what happened and create your new life. The fact that you're reading this book means some part of you is ready! It doesn't matter where you are on your journey—whether you're still deep in the grief cave and not even wanting to believe there is light yet, or you're ready to poke your head out and take a look at the path ahead of you.

You are here and you are precious, lovable and loving, and worthy—even obligated—to live a full life. By reading this book, you're already proving that you care enough about yourself to focus on your self-care and give yourself the necessary tools to navigate this difficult time.

You've got this! Let's begin.

PART 1
THE GRIEF CAVE

Taking Care of Your Body by Gathering Supplies

In the days right after Glen died, I did only what was absolutely necessary, and sometimes not even that. It took weeks before I could properly eat, sleep, and had enough energy just to manage the most pressing estate matters. I didn't go back to work as a coach or teach yoga for almost six weeks, and when I did, it was very part-time and exhausting. I hardly knew how to get out of bed and pick out something to wear; helping others was beyond my ability.

I refer to this time as being in the grief cave. I was disoriented and didn't really know who I was or where I was in my life. I couldn't do even the minor assessment practices I offered in the introductions. All I knew was that I hated what had happened. I was in deep suffering and wanted only one thing—for Glen not to have died. I railed against the universe. I cried and agonized. Part of me knew he was gone and not coming back. But even though I had seen his body, another part of me would not stop thinking he was going to walk around the corner at any moment and tell me it had all been a terrible practical joke.

Years later, I learned through studying grief that not only is this a normal reaction, but it is actually common. Our brains are wired with patterns of familiarity, so looking for your spouse or partner, thinking you might have seen them on the street—these experiences are all perfectly and terribly normal. If only I'd had someone to tell me that I wasn't going crazy in those days, it would have been so comforting!

You are not crazy. You are in grief.

If you're like me, you'll find the grief cave a very uncomfortable place to be and want to get out of it as soon as possible. But we must move carefully. My haphazard escape route—drugs and other irresponsible behaviors—left me in an even deeper hole within the grief cave. Those short-term, pain-relieving behaviors

were, in reality, setbacks—additional obstacles I added to my own healing journey. To get out of the cave and onto my healing path, I had to learn to manage addiction and start prioritizing my health.

The grief cave is a temporary landing place, but you are in charge of how long you stay there. Your friends, family, and coworkers may be ready for you to step out weeks, months, or even years before you are ready, but this is an opportunity to exercise control over your new life. If a well-meaning friend invites you to a gathering and you're not ready to leave the house, that's up to you. Forcing a smile to make others comfortable is not helping anyone and certainly not supporting your healing. You will go when you are ready, and only you know when that is.

In addition to the assessments in the introductions, I invite you to take a moment to observe the tools and supplies you already have piled against the walls of your grief cave. It's possible they are not quite in your view at the moment, but the light of observation may bring them into focus.

When I was in the grief cave, I had the tools of yoga, yoga therapy, and meditation, but I was incapable of using any of them. After one minute in my yoga studio, the silence was so frightening I could only collapse into tears. I was not ready to begin to heal until almost a year later. What made this situation worse was that I was so hard on myself about it. My negative self-talk—*You are a yoga teacher and a coach and a complete mess!*—added to my suffering.

You may have already found that others can add to your suffering as well. There is a future section of the book to help you organize your social connections mindfully. I have also written a complementary book, *Supporting a Survivor of Spouse or Partner Suicide Loss*, that you can give to your friends who want to help but don't know how. As you look around your grief cave and

assess what tools and supports you have to begin your journey, start with the tool of self-support. Here are some possible affirmations you can use when the voice of blame and shame in your head starts to take over or when a misguided friend tells you it's "time to be over it!":

- "I'm grieving."

- "I'm doing my best."

- "I am in the process of healing and recreating my life, and it's hard."

- "I will go at whatever pace feels right for my unique journey."

Your health may not be something you're focusing on right now, but if you want to get moving on your healing journey, a healthy focus can be a huge boost. This includes taking care of your body, your mind, your emotions, and your spiritual life. Each healthy choice you make will strengthen you and remove obstacles to your healing.

The science of yoga, Ayurveda, is the most ancient form of health care. For thousands of years, it has taught us what modern scientific research is now proving—that what the mind experiences, the body experiences. They are connected. A healthy, strong body will improve overall health and well-being and your ability to navigate the rough terrain ahead.

The practices I offer throughout this book are designed to help you connect your body, mind, and emotions and integrate them so you can begin healing. Sometimes when you have experienced trauma, it still resides in your body, so a particular practice may not work. If you feel activated or overwhelmed to the point that you cannot do the practices, I suggest you focus on your breath, take a walk, or connect with a friend. Until you are ready to swim, metaphorically, you may only be able to dip

a toe in the water before you have to back off to what feels safe. Be aware of how you're feeling, and if you begin to feel unsafe or overwhelmed, take care of yourself and leave the practice for now. The point is to heal and recover, not retraumatize yourself.

There are four supplies you will need to use in the grief cave to prepare you for your journey to healing. Let's get started.

You Can Breathe

The rhythm of your breathing will support you through the rest of your life. It seems simple. I mean, of course, you are breathing. It's the first thing you did when you were born, and you've been doing it successfully ever since.

There is an expression "as easy as breathing," but I'm guessing that breathing has not been all that easy for you recently.

Our breath mirrors our feelings. In the weeks and months immediately after Glen died, I frequently found myself panting and gasping for air between sobs and suffering from shallow, stressed breaths during anxiety and panic attacks. I was "F.I.N.E."—Freaked out, Insecure, Neurotic, and Emotional—not the kind of fine I wanted to be. I felt like I was suffocating.

When you feel like you can't breathe, everything becomes difficult and scary. When you learn ways to control your breath—slow it down and regulate it—you'll feel more in control. I know it may seem impossible right now, but I want to assure you: breathing is exactly what you need to do. Really, it's the only thing you need to do immediately.

The first step to reassuring your nervous system that you're okay, that there's no imminent bear attack, is to learn to calm your breathing. I understand this is not easy when you're upset, and I bet you're tired of hearing people tell you to just take a deep breath. That's because when your nervous system thinks a bear

is coming to eat you, taking a deep breath is nearly impossible. Your wiring is set to hyperventilate. Trauma causes long-term stimulation of the nervous system's natural lifesaving response when we don't need it and leads to emotional or physical disease. The good news is you can learn skills to help control this response and allow your body and mind to heal.

Deep, slow breathing regulates your nervous system and reassures your body that it's okay, so digestion, immune function, good cardiovascular function, and sleep can be supported. To get your health back, or to stay as healthy as possible if you haven't gotten sick, find a way to get your breath under control. I know this is a lot to ask, but I'm going to encourage you to try several different techniques until you find one that works for you. There's a reason I've put this skill (oxygen supply) first in this book. It's that important.

The more you practice calming your breath, the faster you will feel better. Breathing well and being aware of your breath is the most effective and useful tip I can give you. Breathing effectively to calm down is not something you have to spend years mastering. The simple breathing techniques I'm going to share with you can make a gigantic difference in how you feel. You will feel stronger, have increased calm and clarity, and be more ready to respond to this unbelievably difficult time.

A Guide to Increase Calm and Clarity by Breathing

Start with one breath. Just take one long, slow deep breath—in and out through your nose. If you can do that, then you can do anything. The breathing techniques I share here are the ones I find the easiest and most calming. There are literally hundreds of breathing techniques available for you to try. Be very careful to

choose one that doesn't make you feel more anxious. Only you can determine if a breathing technique is right for you. If you're going to try techniques other than what I list here and you look them up on the internet, make sure the breathing technique is clearly labeled as "calming" or "restful" or "mindful."

Breathing Positions and Best Practices

There's no striving for mastery here. If you get one long, slow deep breath in, you're doing great. Maybe you can do two next time, and tomorrow, even four or five. Your practice will build on itself; as your mind and emotions feel calmer, breathing will get easier.

The following practices can be done sitting up. If you choose a seated position, place both feet firmly on the floor, gently lengthen your spine, and refrain from leaning against the back of your chair.

You can also lie down. If you're in bed and it's one of those days when getting up seems impossible, stay there. Remember, be gentle with your brain and body. Try to find ease with yourself and don't be hard on yourself for needing a grief day. I used to call my difficult days *wet days*—days when I felt like crying most of the day. I still have them occasionally. Releasing emotions this way, without feeling guilty or trying to stop them, is soothing and healthy. In fact, one of my mentors says that tears are an expression of being deeply connected to yourself. Did you know that crying is a form of extended exhale breath? We'll get to that in a bit.

It's best to close your eyes during breathing practices so you can more completely focus on your breathing and not what you're seeing, but if you're uncomfortable with closing your eyes, try to

look with a soft and unfocused gaze at something just beyond your nose.

Breathe slowly in and out through your nose unless I suggest otherwise. If you're congested, of course you can breathe through your mouth.

Practice 1
Belly Breathing

Place your hands on your lower belly.

As you breathe in, feel your belly expand in all directions, even sideways, and into your back.

As you exhale, gently pull your belly muscles toward your spine.

Keep your shoulders and jaw relaxed as you continue to breathe in and out slowly and deeply.

You can place the tip of your tongue on the spot where your top front teeth meet your gums. This helps remind your jaw to stay relaxed.

Start with three to five breaths and work your way up to five minutes.

Take time after you complete this practice to notice how you feel. Be sure you feel more calm, clear, and centered. If not—if this breath technique makes you feel anxious—then try another one or something different altogether from a different chapter.

All these supplies are meant as support. If it doesn't feel supportive, don't do it!

Practice 2
Elongating the Exhale

In this practice, you will continue deep belly breathing but lengthen the exhale to be longer than the inhale.

Start by taking a few belly breaths as described above, and then count with the natural rhythm of your breath, assigning a number to your inhale and exhale. Whatever number you come up with is fine.

Once you have a number (let's say it's five), after your next inhale, try slowing down your exhale so it takes a count of seven or even eight. Stretch the exhale out so the same amount of air is coming out all throughout the exhale and you don't run out the last few counts.

Ultimately, if you can double the length of the exhale, that's ideal, but simply lengthening the exhale by even one count is effective.

Keep your body and shoulders relaxed. If you start to feel dizzy, breathless, anxious, or light-headed, return to your normal breathing.

Be gentle with yourself; do what works for you.

Practice 3
Hug Breath

The hug breath is the one I use the most when I'm feeling anxious and out of control. Hugs from a caring person can be very healing and can help reset your nervous system. If no one is around to hug you when you need it, or anytime you want to feel cared for and loved, this is the breathing practice for you.

Bring your right hand to your chest over your heart and feel your heartbeat. Keep your shoulder relaxed and just bend your elbow.

Bring your left hand to your lower belly and feel the deep, calming belly breaths.

This may be enough to calm you, but I want to suggest you add a mantra here. When I do this, I repeat to myself, silently or out loud, "I am safe. I am safe. I am safe."

This practice got me through many middle-of-the-night freak attacks when no one was around to hug or talk to. You can use any words that feel comforting to you, perhaps "I am loved," or "I am okay," or "I will survive." Mantras and affirmations are very helpful for increasing the effectiveness of breathing practices, and I'll share more on that later.

Breathing techniques are extremely powerful, but only choose one that makes you feel better. It may take a few tries to find one that makes you feel calmer and more in control. Try out a new practice slowly and for just a few minutes to start. Then check in with yourself and see how you feel. If the breathing technique you tried made you feel more anxious, try another one. If one works particularly well, make a note of it, so it's easy to remember to use when you need it.

Fuel Your Journey

It can be difficult to sit at the table where you shared so many meals with your spouse or partner, let alone think about food. Thinking about Glen's favorite meal and seeing his food in the pantry—it broke my heart so many times. I found eating in a different room helped. Take-out meals also allowed me to avoid cooking in the kitchen, where we shared so many memories. It helped me to eat foods we had never shared and to try completely new recipes—things that only appealed to me, even things I knew he would have hated. If you are able to get out of the house, go eat at a friend's place whenever possible. Your friends want to support you; however, they often need to be educated on how to support you. Ask them to invite you over for a meal and even to make extra that you can take home for another meal, so you don't have to cook. They will be relieved that they are doing something to help you. I know that's only a short-term solution, but it can be helpful to separate eating, which is an absolutely necessary activity, from painful memories and grief.

There are a lot of things that are more than unusual right now in your life. Eating may be on that list. You may be overeating high-fat, high-calorie foods, stress eating, or not eating at all. Whatever is going on, be gentle with yourself; this is not the time to berate yourself for that extra cookie or midnight pizza. It is important, however, to nourish yourself the best you can. It's

possible you've been able to continue eating and digesting food as you always did, depending on your gut health and the strength of your digestion going into this crisis. Some people will use food as a source of comfort. If this is you, don't beat yourself up. For now, that's okay! If you're like me, however, you will struggle to swallow or digest anything while you're in shock and grieving. Not only was I not hungry during the time around Glen's death, but even when I tried to eat, I could hardly make enough saliva to get anything from my mouth to my stomach. Stress completely shut down my digestion. I could drink—I was a champ at that!—but my diet of coffee and vodka was not helping me gain any strength for my healing journey.

If you're having trouble with your digestion, just take it slow. Remember earlier when I was describing what's going on with your body under stress? Your traumatized nervous system may have shut down your digestion because your body is preparing to fight or flee from the bear. Even if it seems almost impossible, it's more important now than ever to give your body the best nutrition you can. Emotional recovery and physical recovery go hand in hand, so try to take care of your body by eating nourishing food.

But how can you possibly eat well when you feel so terrible? Here are a few ideas that will help:

1. **Sit quietly, take a deep breath, and think about your favorite foods.** Focus as much as possible on the details of how the food tastes, its smell and textures, and perhaps your stomach will start churning, beginning the digestive process by releasing enzymes that will help you feel hungry and then break down your food. When you feel hungry, eat nutritious food if you can; if not, just eat!

2. **Be mindful but not picky.** If *any* food sounds good, even french fries, get them and eat them. Milkshakes and soups worked well for me because I had so little in the way of digestive juices, so liquid-based foods were good (but avoid too much caffeine or alcohol). Protein shakes are good too, and there are some with low sugar and good nutrition in them!

3. **Get as much variety as possible.** Obviously, this isn't a time to go on any type of diet, but do pay attention to what you're putting in your body. If eggs sound good, great! Eat eggs. But try not to eat *only* eggs if you can help it. Throw in some toast or maybe some avocado. Remember, you need protein, fats, and fiber together to get the nutrition you need. If you can only eat eggs, or pizza, at least you're eating! And eating is necessary for your healing journey.

4. **Get your digestion going by drinking eight ounces of warm-to-hot water first thing in the morning and/ or fifteen minutes before each meal.** This helps your stomach lining wake up and secrete digestive enzymes, and in about fifteen to twenty minutes, you may feel hungry and have your stomach ready for food. Digestive aids, such as apple cider vinegar (one tablespoon in eight ounces of water before a meal) or digestive bitters, can also help get your digestion going.

If you aren't eating, or aren't eating anything nutritious, you can consult your doctor or a nutritionist. Your body needs fuel to heal, and what you eat can very much determine how you feel. You'll feel better if you eat better, so keep trying until you find something that works.

Hydration is also very important for healing. If you hate water, then drink sparkling water, or even better, kombucha (look for low sugar), which can support digestion.

Remember, be gentle with yourself and take care, drink water, and eat as well as you can. You'll get through this, and eating well will make it easier.

Rest and Sleep

Sleep was not a thing I could do at all for a long time after Glen died. Those late nights staring at the place he used to occupy in our bed and ruminating about the dreadful times leading up to and after his death kept me awake most nights. Sometimes I would briefly fall asleep and then wake up screaming in terror. Despite the prescribed medications and other drugs I used to try to get sleep, my nights were mostly torture.

It makes sense that you can't just lie down peacefully and enjoy restful sleep when your heart is racing because your nervous system is acting like a bear is chasing you. What I came to realize was that if I wasn't sleeping, everything felt worse. Sleepless nights are like adding another hundred pounds to the backpack you're carrying on your journey. Eventually I learned some practices that worked for sleep, and I began to feel better.

To seek relief, I changed things up. I moved my bed to another wall in the room and got new sheets and a comforter, which helped ease the intensity of those memories.

Sleep has recently entered the scientific literature as a high-impact health practice. Professional athletes have started altering their travel schedules based on getting a full eight hours between contests. Hundreds of studies are out now indicating how important good quality sleep is to your health and well-being. Good sleep has been shown to lower cholesterol, blood pressure,

and blood sugar (keeping diabetes at bay). And of course, you think more clearly, feel happier, and are more energetic when you get good sleep. Sleep supports healing.

You Can Do It!

Sleep is so very essential, and if you prioritize it and focus on it, you can do it! If you were able to start practicing some of the breathing and mindfulness techniques described earlier, your sleep may have already improved. When you're wide awake in the middle of the night, instead of reaching for your phone, a breathing practice or meditation practice can offer comfort and calm and support more restful sleep.

You are probably aware of how important sleep is, but you may not know how to get any restful sleep when you're suffering. You may be using late-night drinking, other substances, unhealthy eating (who is going to make a superfood smoothie at midnight? Bring on the ice cream!), or TV to self-soothe during those miserable hours instead of getting proper sleep. Let me reinforce for you that if you prioritize sleep and bring good sleep hygiene into your life, the lonely late nights and the difficult foggy days will improve much faster.

Sleep and Digestion

Digestion refers to more than just what you eat and drink. We also have to digest all of our experiences from the day. Deep sleep is where your brain has a chance to digest emotions and experiences from each day. For physical and emotional health reasons, we need to give our bodies time and support for digestion.

If you are up late watching disturbing news programs or horror movies, you are doing yourself a disservice. The early hours of the night, between 10 p.m. and 2 a.m., are very important for brain/emotional cleansing. And everything you "ingest," from food to everything you watch on TV, every conversation you have, and every thought and experience you have during the day, needs to be processed—digested. You are already under enough stress right now; give yourself the best chance to heal and recover by avoiding anything that might be unnecessarily stressful or upsetting, especially near bedtime.

Soon after Glen died, I found myself watching the Disney movies I used to enjoy with my kids when they were little. They were all I could handle. They held my attention and, for a brief time, gave me a respite from terror. The less stress, the better. Comedy is great. If you can find anything to make you laugh, you are helping yourself to heal. I love musicals, cat videos, and movies with lots of beautiful music and scenery.

You may love horror movies or movies with a lot of violence, but your brain has to work really hard to cleanse and process all those intense images. Exposing yourself to unhealthy food and beverages or toxic movies and shows is like adding to your already-too-heavy backpack. Give your body and emotions a break by finding something light to ingest.

Sleep and Drugs

After Glen died, I was suffering so deeply I was open to just about anything anyone suggested that might take the edge off or help me find a way out of the agony that was the reality of my life. My doctor prescribed everything she thought could give me some relief. Some of the drugs helped temporarily, but nothing actually

worked for any length of time, and usually I felt worse when the effects wore off. In trauma therapy, I learned that many drugs and medications can contribute to depression or delay emotional processing, so please talk to your doctor and take only what you absolutely need to help you for the immediate future.

For months after Glen's death, I tried to escape my pain by drinking, smoking, and using various drugs. Well-meaning friends brought me every imaginable drug—over the counter, prescription, and illegal.

Smoking cigarettes, I rationalized, was something I *could* do; and when disabled by grief, anything I could *do* felt like an accomplishment. Plus, I thought they helped calm me. FYI: nicotine is a stimulant and does *not* calm you. The only thing that might be beneficial is the presence involved in smoking. Going outside and taking deep breaths (if you smoke, you know it is an extended exhale, like a sigh) can seem calming, but if you're looking for a truly calming experience, find a breath practice and do it without the toxins and nicotine.

Besides smoking a ridiculous number of cigarettes, I drank a lot of vodka, and then I added, among other things, weed, Xanax, antidepressants, and cocaine. I really got into trouble.

About seven months after Glen died, I was so sick from all the chemicals I was putting into my body, while also not eating and sleeping, that a very good friend of mine threatened to put me into rehab. This shocked me. Even though I had just confessed to him all the details of the substances I was misusing and depending on to ease my suffering, I couldn't imagine I was addicted and needed to go to a program to get clean. I was just trying to get through every day. But my friend was very serious, and that threat was enough to get me to take a hard look at myself. My friend also strongly encouraged me to start trauma therapy, which I did.

I couldn't believe it when even my trauma therapist told me that no amount of the self-prescribed mind- and body-numbing substances I was taking was okay *if my goal was healing*. I started bargaining. "What if I just do this stuff on the weekends? That's surely okay." She explained how taking drugs to numb myself was not only lowering my resilience and causing me to be sick all the time, but it was interfering with and delaying any chance I had to recover, heal, and create my new life. Deep inside, I was miserable enough to know she was right.

I'm not telling you to quit all the self-soothing chemicals and unhealthy habits you may have right now, especially if, for instance, taking sleeping pills is the only way you can get sleep. Your use of substances and weaning off of them needs to be a slow, careful process done with the help of your doctor and therapist, so you don't get worse before you get better. Just keep in mind that long-term, unhealthy choices only add weight to your backpack, making your journey to recreate your life an even harder climb.

Guide to Sleeping Well

You may be sleeping more or less than usual at this time. Sleep is really vital for healing, so try to get at least *some* sleep when you can. I realize some of the sleep tips I'm sharing are going to sound nearly impossible, especially if you've never had an easy time sleeping. But if you can shift into healthy sleeping habits, not only will your backpack lighten, your recovery will be easier, and your entire life will improve! Just look through and see if any of these practices seem possible to try. As always, they are only suggestions. Do what you can, and try not to be hard on yourself!

Practice 1
Go to bed at the same time every night.

If you get into a rhythm, your body will get used to knowing it's lights-out time. Limit exposure to screens before bed. For example, if right now you're watching TV until 3 a.m., tonight, turn off the TV at 2 a.m. and read something boring or inspiring (not a horror novel) or listen to soothing music. If it doesn't work tonight, just keep trying. You can always try the breathing techniques to fill the time until sleep comes. If you regularly fall asleep at 2 a.m., slowly, fifteen minutes per night, move your sleep schedule to 10 p.m. The ideal sleep schedule for most humans is approximately 10 p.m. to 6 a.m. Some of us need more than eight hours of sleep. Once you get yourself back to being able to sleep regularly, your body will tell you how much sleep you need. Imagine waking up feeling rested and refreshed! It *is* possible. We are not nocturnal creatures, so if you synchronize your sleep schedule with natural rhythms, you will improve your health and well-being.

Practice 2
Eat earlier in the evening.

For sleep to be the most cleansing and supportive to your brain, your body needs to focus its energetic processes on digesting the emotional experiences from the day, not the food you ate right before bed. Finish eating two to three hours before you try to sleep. Again, take it slow. I used to fall asleep with a half-drunk vodka next to my bed. If you're used to drinking alcohol or eating a late-night snack in bed, exchange it for warm milk or water,

and maybe add a tablespoon of turmeric and some honey. This is called golden milk, and it can be very soothing before bed.

Practice 3
Wake up in the morning without an alarm.

Yes, I know that sounds crazy, but if you go to bed early and sleep deeply, you will wake feeling refreshed and ready for your day. Of course, this can vary widely during an intense period of grief and loss. Remember, even if you feel like you haven't done much today, you are putting tremendous effort into healing right now, so you may feel exhausted. If you find yourself sleeping twelve hours per night and wanting naps too, please do that. Any sleep you can get is healing! Be gentle with yourself. If your body says rest and you possibly can, do it.

Practice 4
Don't nap.

Naps are a little controversial in the literature. Some sleep experts recommend them, some don't. Ayurveda, the ancient health science that informs my work, does not recommend napping. If you feel so tired at midday that a nap (or a double espresso) is the only way you feel you can cope, then please nap and skip the espresso. Try to make it twenty minutes to an hour at the most. This way, you will get a little refreshed without interfering with your much-needed deep sleep at night. Again, these are tips for long-term, ideal sleep hygiene. Right now, when you are in grief, any sleep you can get at any time is awesome.

Practice 5
Establish a bedtime routine to help your body get into a pattern of knowing when it's time to sleep.

Here are some good practices for a bedtime routine:

1. Shut down all screens an hour before sleep.

2. Keep your room cool and dark.

3. Take a shower or bath and/or rub soothing warm oil on your feet, using a scent you like that is calming, like lavender or chamomile.

4. Journal at bedtime. This can be a great way to begin the transition to sleep. Writing (on paper if possible, not on your phone, which counts as a screen) five things you are grateful for about your day can really help you settle your emotions and improve your mood. Writing about your day helps jumpstart the cleansing process your brain will need to go through, mostly during sleep, for optimal health. Begin by writing the last thing you did: "I lay down on my bed." Or you can be less specific: "I got ready for bed." Then go backward through your day, listing what you did, how you felt about the experiences you had, and finally, end with what time you woke up and how you slept. Then, set an intention for how you will sleep tonight: "I will have a deep, restful sleep." You can even write that a few times.

5. If you're not sleepy yet, turn on some music or perhaps a guided meditation. This is also a great time to do a body scan meditation to see how you're feeling and release any tension you find. (Check out Part 2 for this meditation.)

I know this sounds like a lot, and it would be very difficult to do all of this if your current bedtime routine is eating pizza and drinking alcohol late at night until you pass out. I get it. I did that for a long time. And, I was able to shift very slowly by adding one practice at a time, cutting down on my late-night pizza and vodka, and increasing my awareness of how I felt when I woke up after going to bed earlier and using fewer substances. I felt a lot better. Take all the time you need. Pick one or two practices and see how it goes.

And if you just can't do anything on this list right now, so be it. Be gentle with yourself. Eventually, when you feel ready to try to prioritize sleep, you can try these practices.

Move to Heal

Before Glen died, I had been an active person. As a yoga therapist, a personal trainer, and a former athlete, I was well-acquainted, through education and personal experience, with the health benefits of movement. In the weeks following Glen's death, however, I spent almost all my time sitting in bed or behind my house drinking, smoking, and crying. On top of the emotional pain, my physical body hurt, and any attempt at yoga ended in tears.

I felt heavier and heavier. And even though I knew my lack of movement was adding to my feelings of depression, anxiety and fatigue, stuckness, stiffness, and soreness, I just couldn't get myself to move. The weight of the grief, trauma, and shock buried me; it was too much to bear. It was as if when the ground disappeared beneath me, I knocked loose an avalanche of rubble that tumbled down on top of me.

Movement is another basic staple of well-being. Moving your body helps you feel better. Physical movement can help get those emotions flowing and processing. That includes moving the emotions out from where they're stuck in your body and releasing them. If you already have movement in your life, perhaps you were able to keep going with your regular exercise routine or you returned to it before this book came into your world. That's great! Keep moving and caring for your health by doing so.

Move Mindfully

Movement is so important and necessary for our health. If you can get your body moving, even for ten minutes each day, you will begin to feel better. If you don't feel like you have ten minutes, check out the four-minute practice to challenge every major muscle group in your body created by Zach Bush, MD, a wonderful resource for health, nutrition, and healing our world.[3]

To mindfully improve your recovery, try to connect to your body and emotions and surroundings at least once during your exercise time. Just for a moment, check in with yourself: How do you feel right now? If you're lucky enough to be outside, connect your awareness to the nature that surrounds you. Can you hear birds or see other animals or something green? Adding mindful presence to your movement can keep you in tune with how you're feeling, so you can feel the flow of healing traveling through you.

This is one of the benefits of yoga. Yoga incorporates mindful movement and breathing practices all into one activity, so you can deeply tune in to how you are feeling and, with that awareness, find the tools you need to move through your recovery.

If you aren't an exerciser at all, that's okay. There are lots of ways to add movement into your life. Maybe you listen to a podcast while you run, or watch an enjoyable show while on the treadmill, or dance to your favorite music. Whatever movement you are doing is great. Just figure out what works for you and add this new habit slowly; make it doable.

You can begin by taking a walk outside. If you live near a park or can easily drive to one, then get yourself there. Studies show being in nature is good for your health, so you are being healthy in two ways: moving your body *and* connecting with nature. By connecting, I don't mean you have to hug a tree or walk barefoot

in the dirt (although these are nourishing practices if you feel up to it!); just use your senses to be fully present.

Perhaps getting outside feels like too much right now. Okay, then I invite you to put this book down and stand up. Raise your hands over your head and stretch to the right and left, bend forward a bit, then sit back down and congratulate yourself. If you can add a bit more movement each day, you will begin to get your body flowing, and your mind and emotions will follow. Stuckness anywhere in the mind, emotions, or body adds more weight to your backpack and makes it a more difficult climb.

If you have a supportive friend who does a movement form you enjoy or think you might enjoy, ask them to include you. Maybe it's a class at their gym or a walk with them around their neighborhood, so then you're getting social time *and* movement! Bonus! Just be sure it's someone who knows you need support and that this is part of your healing—someone who will help you unpack a little bit from your backpack along the way.

Also, there are so many online classes now. If you aren't up for leaving the house, set up an exercise spot near a window you can open for fresh air and find something you like to do. Then do it!

If you can get regular movement into your life, whether it's a new habit or you've been a lifelong exerciser, you will strengthen yourself in body, mind, and emotions, and this difficult time will become lighter and easier.

Congratulations on completing Part 1. With your new and remembered tools, you may now be ready to step out of the grief cave. Only you can decide when you're ready to move or change anything about your life. Perhaps it's enough just knowing you have hope of someday using your tools to improve how you feel and help you heal. Every step on your healing journey is up to you, and when you are ready, there's more support for your growth and healing ahead in Part 2.

PART 2
THE REST STOPS

Releasing Mental and Emotional Burdens

Stepping out of the grief cave and beginning your new life can be whatever you experience it to be. You may go to a movie or the grocery store and find that the "normal" people doing "normal" things is comforting, or it could just be too much. I remember one of my first trips to the grocery store after Glen died. When the checker simply asked how my day was going, I burst into tears. I wasn't ready to deal with someone asking me how I was doing.

You may discover that you only want to interact with people who understand grief and loss and suicide. Hopefully you have found a supportive therapist or coach. There are also communities online you can reach out to for this type of support. Stick with people and activities that feel supportive and leave the rest for now.

This is your journey, your climb. It's up to you to choose what supports you. Use what works and release what doesn't.

Leaving the cave, your pack may be full of helpful supplies for your journey. But as you take those first few tentative steps, you may find that you need to readjust the weight and unpack some of the burdens you didn't previously see in that backpack of yours. In this next part, you'll have the opportunity to unload what is not supporting your journey. You'll find useful supplies (stay tuned for how to use the candle, notebook or journal, phone, and matches), but you may also find heavy burdens (who put the rock in my backpack?!) that need to be released as you journey toward healing. In fact, with every step you take at first, you'll likely ask, "What is making this so hard?" When this happens, it's time to pull off the path for a rest stop, set down the backpack, take a rest, and reassess. Find what is burdensome and release it.

Take as many rests as you need, including days when you feel like crawling all the way back into the grief cave and recharging. The cave won't be the same as it was those first weeks and months

because your journey to healing has begun. Even if you haven't done any of the practices in Part 1, simply being able to say "It's been two months" instead of "It's been two days" means there has been a change. Time has passed, and although I don't believe time alone can heal, it does cause change.

> **Mindfulness practices are the most effective way to release burdens and gain control of your feelings and the best tool I can offer to support you to move along this journey toward healing.**

Just before Glen died, he emptied our joint bank account and opened a new one in his name only. This made it impossible for me to pay my bills. I discovered this when I got a message from the bank saying I was overdrawn. I quickly had to assess my options, figure out where I was financially, and get help to cover as many of my bills as possible. Step one here was assessing my resources. (Well, to be honest, step one was me getting really angry at him, which of course, did not pay the bills.) I asked a few friends for temporary loans, and I was able to draw some equity from my house.

But in order to figure these things out, I had to stop and breathe and reassure myself I was okay (even if I was sure I was not okay) so I could think clearly enough to decide which bills to pay first. I used the exact techniques I described in Part 1 and then the ones here to meet this challenge and the hurdles that showed up next.

Help yourself confront your mountain of challenges—emotional, physical, relational, financial, or some combination—by adding mindfulness to your toolbox.

This is an extremely difficult time, but if you can develop some mindful awareness of yourself and your circumstances, it will lessen your suffering. Your journey to healing will be a

smoother, easier climb. Your backpack will be lighter, and you'll be more able to catch yourself when the path leads you away from your goal or if some unexpected challenge causes you to fall into a temporary slide.

Mindfulness is about being aware of the present moment without judging it or trying to change it. If you have a moment of mindful, nonjudgmental awareness or presence, you are, in that moment, not suffering. And if you get even a few of those each day, your burden will lighten tremendously. You will be more calm and clear, and your body will know, at least for a time, that you are not being chased by a bear.

I remember sitting in my backyard and yelling at the universe the day after Glen died. When I heard myself say, "And now I'm a widow," my rant stopped abruptly. Those five words took my breath away. More than that temporary realization of the situation stopped me: I had pulled something out of the chaos of shock and disbelief of this unreal situation—something that was true—and, at least for a second, I accepted that truth.

For days after Glen died, I was a complete mess. I hadn't eaten or slept, and I'd been on the phone or had visitors every moment I wasn't in bed. I was sure I was dreaming and that I would wake up from the nightmare at any moment.

I was completely overwhelmed.

On day three or four, I had another moment of not feeling completely out of control—a moment of presence. It didn't last long, but it was a welcome respite from the horror I was living. I was washing my hands. The simple act of washing hands doesn't seem like a big moment of relief, but this was powerful because I was present for it. Suddenly, the complete chaos I'd been living in within my mind became still as I focused intently on the water and the soap and watched the bubbles reflect the light making rainbows. I felt the temperature and the softness of the water and

my hands rubbing together. I smelled the beautiful scent of the lavender in the soap. This experience of presence lasted only a few seconds, but it was the first moment since I had found Glen's body that I was able to actually be where I was. This moment of mindfulness gave me a break from rampaging thoughts and emotions, and for just a fleeting moment, I experienced peace.

A Guide to Being

It takes effort to cultivate a practice that allows you to be where you are, but the benefits of mindfulness are absolutely worth the effort.

Being can be a difficult practice, but it is second only to *breathing* as far as the impact it can have on your state of mind. There is a difference between suffering from anxiety, grief, sorrow, trauma, and anger and being aware that you are anxious, grieving, sad, traumatized, and angry. This difference impacts where your pain level is—it's the difference between struggling up a steep rocky trail or walking easily through your journey. Instead of your emotions controlling you, you cultivate the practice of being with them: "I feel anger" instead of "I am angry." Once you become *aware* of how you feel, instead of *suffering from* how you feel, you will have increased your capacity to respond with kindness to your emotions rather than react in a way you may regret. You can pick out a tool to use to help you feel better.

Mindfulness brings acceptance. You can't change the past, and you can't control the future.

The past can't be changed, and the future cannot be controlled, but you *can* change how you feel about it all if you are mindfully present. I know how hard that can be. I desperately wished I could

go back and change the past, and I was terrified of my future after Glen's death. I wanted so desperately for things to be different than they were. This wanting only made things worse. It took a lot of work, but when I accepted the fact that what happened *had happened*, and no matter how much I wanted to, *I could not change the past*, my backpack became significantly lighter.

What we resist persists.
Resisting what is increases suffering.

The stages of grief, developed from theories about the process of dying by Elizabeth Kubler-Ross and adapted to the process of grieving by her and David Kessler, are anger, denial, bargaining, depression, and acceptance. Later, David Kessler added a sixth stage: finding meaning. The stages are not experienced in any particular order, and once you've been in one, you may revisit it many times. Eventually, you'll go through them and process them, and they will not cause as much suffering because you'll recognize them when they happen. Mindfully recognizing the feelings, the grief stage you are in, will allow you to feel more in control. Noticing *I'm feeling anger right now*, instead of being consumed by the feeling, will keep you moving forward on your journey. You can be in any stage at any time. There is no wrong, and you won't be there forever. Mindfully noticing the stage can be very supportive during your journey.

Separating Story from Feeling

Did you know you have 60,000 to 80,000 thoughts per day? And did you know that almost all these thoughts are the same ones you had yesterday? The intensity of the experience you are in right now will probably make that easy to grasp. You probably

go to sleep with your challenging, racing thoughts and wake up with those same thoughts. When I work with clients who are experiencing grief, we always do a thought awareness practice that helps to make these runaway thoughts manageable.

The thoughts are your story. Some are true and some may be conclusions your mind has drawn about your spouse's death and what caused it that may or may not be true. (Especially if you're blaming yourself—that one is not true.) The practice I'm offering here is to notice when you are racing around in your story and then have the presence to come back to the current moment.

When we are in grief, we can get caught up in our story and not realize that it is just that—our story—and that, just like a book, we can put it down when we need a break. Mindfulness practices allow us to do that. Those racing thoughts that keep you up in the middle of the night, and possibly terrorize you all day, can be softened, slowed, and even stopped.

When I ask my clients, "How are you feeling?" many immediately launch into their story, recounting all the terrible thoughts they're having that are causing suffering. I listen patiently (because that's the number one thing we grievers need—witnessing) and then ask again, "How are you feeling right now?" Eventually, when they're ready, I give them an assignment to notice how they are feeling. Connecting to your feelings is one of the most important parts of healing. Stepping out of the terrible story you keep retelling and noticing how you are feeling—noticing that the feeling isn't always connected to or even related to the story. I invite you to practice this the next time someone asks you how you are doing. Instead of launching into stories about what happened when your partner died, what's going on with the estate, who in your world isn't behaving the way you wish they would, or what you can or cannot accept right now, take a breath and really deeply feel. How are you *feeling*

right now—in this moment? Just exploring that will give you a break from your story. Each time you give yourself that break and notice you are doing it, you are adding another powerful tool to your healing toolbox.

Meditation, a form of mindfulness, helps you manage what you think. With practice, you can actually choose what you think about. Imagine, you're watching TV and all you can think about is the last time you watched this show with your late husband. Or you think you need to have another drink or smoke or pill to make it through the next few minutes, days, weeks. Or you can't stop thinking about that horribly insensitive comment your well-meaning friend made that actually made you feel worse than you have in days. Or you're up at 2 a.m., worried sick because you don't know how you're going to pay your bills. If you stop, let that thought go, and choose a different one, you are taking control instead of allowing the thoughts to control you. Then maybe you can turn to another thought—like remembering when you watched that movie and he leaned over and gave you that magical kiss? You can trade thoughts of loss for thoughts of love, like the feeling of that kiss and, for a moment, remember the love you shared. Meditation can help you feel the kiss of love more than the pain of loss. With practice, you can actually choose to think thoughts that bring joy and love.

Mindful Presence and Being Practices

You can choose to be mindful at any moment—bringing yourself into the present, connecting with your physical body—and this will stop your spiraling emotions, bring you calm and peace, and center you. It's just a matter of practice. If you are practicing any of the breathing techniques, you already have a mindfulness practice. Those techniques are mindful breathing!

Here are some more accessible mindfulness practices to try that may help you find some relief when you are suffering.

Mindfulness Practice 1
The Five Senses

Sit comfortably with your feet on the floor and interlace your fingers or bring your palms together at your heart in any hand position that feels stabilizing. If you're really agitated, you can do this standing, walking, or wherever you are (except while driving).

1. **See:** Look around. Notice five things you can see in your environment. Don't judge or react ("Oh, I meant to clean that up," or "Wow, I need to dust that"). Just note them. Observe them with your eyes as if you've never seen them before, and if you feel the urge, name them silently to yourself.

2. **Hear:** Close your eyes or lower your gaze and listen. List four things you can hear. Take a few minutes if you need to. You may only hear a couple of things. It's not the achievement of a goal but the practice of focusing your attention that supports you. And if there's an annoying noise, like your neighbor's barking dog or a loud TV, listen for the spaces *between* the noise.

3. **Feel:** List three things you can feel with your senses. It may be the fabric of your clothes, the chair you are resting on, or your hands and fingers. Remember, there's no right or wrong; just try to focus your attention.

4. **Smell:** Inhale and try to detect the aroma of two things. You may be able to smell more or fewer. Don't worry. Just focus on your sense of smell for a minute or so.

5. **Taste:** What do you taste right now? Usually, even if you haven't eaten or had anything to drink recently, there is still a sense of taste you can experience and name.

Now, notice how you feel. Hopefully, you are feeling calmer and more in tune with yourself. If not, repeat the process after taking a few deep belly breaths.

Mindfulness Practice 2
Connect with the Earth

Sit or lie down. Take some slow deep breaths, and then focus your attention anywhere your body is touching a surface. Notice your hands in your lap, your legs on the chair, your feet on the floor. Keep your attention on these areas and imagine your body connecting energetically through the chair, through the floor, and through the foundation of the building you're in, as if you're growing roots all the way through the earth to its core. The earth is always there for you, supporting and sustaining you. Focus on that connection as long as your attention allows. While you're at it, enjoy a moment of gratitude for gravity!

Mindfulness Practice 3
Sustained Gazing

Use a favorite item—something that brings you joy or is at least neutral. It could be a crystal, any type of stone, or a candle, which can be a great item to practice with because it's constantly moving and changing, making it easier to hold attention. Choose something small enough that you can see the whole thing without moving your eyes. Place the item you choose in front of you, or

maybe in your hands, and take a couple of deep belly breaths. Bring your entire attention to the item. Notice the size, shape, and color. Notice how the light reflects off of it and if it casts a shadow. While you relax your body and keep your breathing deep, continue to look at the item with a soft gaze for as long as you can. The item may seem to waver, grow or shrink, or get darker or lighter. This is all just your eyes reacting to stillness and is nothing to worry about. As always, if this practice is not calming for you, stop and find a different one!

Mindfulness Practice 4
Body Scan

Starting at the top of your head, move your awareness through your body slowly all the way down to the bottoms of your feet. Notice if anything feels tense: your face, or your jaw, your neck, or your shoulders. If you find tension anywhere, focus on a deep belly breath for a moment. Imagine your inhale bringing healing and calm and your exhale releasing tension. Stop anywhere on your body where you don't feel ease, take a deep belly breath, and imagine breathing ease into that area. Breathe out, releasing tension with your exhale. It may take a couple of rounds, but keep it up. Being aware of where you hold tension in your body is a great start to releasing it.

Mindfulness Practice 5
Locating and Naming Emotions in the Body

For every emotion we feel, there is a corresponding physical sensation. Usually, unless you've had trauma therapy, or yoga training, or some other type of emotional awareness training,

you won't notice it. This technique has helped me out of so many difficult moments when I felt my emotions were completely out of control.

The awareness practices I've already discussed will help you to know when you're feeling an uncomfortable emotion. When you notice you're feeling uncomfortable emotions, instead of focusing on the emotion and saying something like, "I am so upset right now, I want to break something!" or "I am so sad right now, I wish I could just melt into this couch and disappear," bring your attention to your body. If you are feeling anxious, perhaps your chest is tight or your tummy is upset.

Concentrate on where the feeling is in your body. For example, *I am feeling anger.* Then, locate where in your body you are feeling the anger. It may be in your stomach, your chest, your throat, or somewhere else. There's no wrong answer here; the practice is understanding how your emotions connect to your body. Once you have that in mind, name where you feel it, maybe even out loud: "I feel this in my chest." Then describe the quality of the feeling if you can. Does it feel hot or cold, tight, prickly, heavy? Give it a try; see if you can feel anything right now.

Once you have identified the physical location of the anger, you can breathe into it and attempt to release it. You can also do specific movements to release emotions from within the physical body. It's just a matter of being present for them and learning the techniques. Earlier, I mentioned that naming an emotion can help you feel more in control. Bringing your awareness to the place in your body where you feel the emotion is another method of diffusing its intensity and helping you gain more control.

Mindfulness Practice 6
Meditation

Meditation can help you manage your thoughts and feelings so your mind doesn't just run wild. When your body thinks you're being chased by a bear, regular meditation can help control the stress reaction and keep it from damaging your health.

It took me a year after Glen died to get back into a regular meditation practice. While I was at the retreat at the Chopra Center in 2017, the meditation practices created a significant, positive emotional shift for me. The twice-daily practice of mantra meditation was part of this retreat. Although it was very challenging to start, eventually it became one of the biggest leaps in my healing journey. Anyone can meditate, so don't believe for a second that just because you don't like to sit still or your mind runs out of control that a meditation practice, and all the benefits that come with it, isn't within your ability.

Meditations

Here are some things to try. If they don't work for you right now, revisit them when you're ready. As I always tell potential students, yoga and meditation will be there for you whenever you are ready to practice.

Meditation Practice 1
Breath Awareness

Sit comfortably with your eyes closed and take deep belly breaths. Notice your breath coming in and out of your nose. Notice how the air coming in is a bit cooler than the air going out. Keep this

up as long as possible, starting with one minute. When you notice thoughts popping in (and they will, and that's perfectly okay), just let them go and return your attention to your breathing. That's it! You just meditated. Not so bad, huh? If this was a good experience for you, try it for an additional minute each day, and aim for ten to twenty minutes of comfortable breath awareness. If it seems impossible, remember even one minute, even one breath, can help break the cycle of suffering from your thoughts.

Meditation Practice 2
Mantra

Translated from Sanskrit (the ancient language of yoga), mantra means "mind tools." These are literally tools to anchor your attention so your mind can be as still as possible. Mantras can be meaningless sounds or very specific words with vibrations designed to give a particular outcome, such as health, love, calm, wealth, peace, or compassion.

You can use any word or phrase that helps your mind stay focused and possibly even calm. The word *OM* (pronounced A-UM) is a great one because as the vibrations resonate, they can help process emotions. Sometimes I use *So Hum*. I like this mantra because I can match the words to my breath: inhale *So*, exhale *Hum*. Shalom and salaam are similar and can feel resonant with peace. You could use "I am safe" or "I am here." If none of these appeal to you, research mantras or choose a word or phrase that feels right for you.

Once you have chosen your mantra, sit comfortably with your eyes closed and repeat the mantra silently to yourself. Whenever you notice your thoughts wandering to sounds in the environment, physical sensations, or anything other than the

mantra, simply and gently return your attention to repeating the mantra. It is this awareness and repeated returning that holds the power of the practice. The mantra may speed up or slow down; it may shift and change in feeling or internal sound. There's no wrong here. Just keep returning your attention to the mantra. Start small, a minute or so, and add a minute each day. Some days will be easier than others; just keep at it. The only way to do meditation wrong is to not do it at all.

When you bring mindfulness and meditation into your life, your suffering will ease. Next time you notice you're feeling guilty for your partner's suicide, or find that you are shoulding on yourself ("I should have . . ." or "I should . . ."), take a moment to breathe. Bring yourself back to the present moment by using one of the practices above. You can even choose a different thought: *I loved my partner and did everything I could*, or *I cannot change what happened*, or *Love lives on*, or any comforting phrase. You deserve to feel supported, especially by you.

Feelings are like a garden—what you nurture is what will grow.

Meditation, this practice of being where you are, is powerful. Think of it as having trekking poles that help you navigate the rougher terrain of your journey. Use these trekking poles to help you balance or as an aid to help you up a steep incline. But just like staying in shape for anything, it takes consistent practice. The more you practice, the stronger you get. It's best to practice daily so you can strengthen the muscle of mindfulness when you aren't in an immediately stressful situation. When faced with a high-stress moment, you will be ready to manage practically any challenging situation.

I have some simple, very doable free meditations on my website and YouTube channel, which you will find in the resources. I can teach you how to meditate and coach you to help make meditation easy and accessible. You can also download some really great apps, such as Insight Timer, Headspace, and the Chopra app. Those apps have a variety of meditations focused on grief, sorrow, and trauma. Just look for one that resonates with you, with someone whose voice you enjoy. There are also calming music tracks on these apps. If you can find music you like, just sit and listen and focus completely on the music.

Start small—one minute at a time, one meditation at a time. If you want to run a marathon (and you are running an emotional marathon right now), you must train for it. Meditation and mindfulness practices increase emotional resilience, make life easier and more joyful, and help ease your healing journey.

Unprocessed Feelings

Emotions need a healthy outlet; they need to go somewhere and be witnessed if they are to be healed. However, there are healthy and unhealthy ways to process emotions. We need to be careful to process emotions in ways that we don't regret and in ways that increase our strength and resilience and don't make us feel worse. Activities like drinking too much, using drugs, breaking things, or alienating loved ones may help us discharge emotions, but they do not further our healing. One of my meditation teachers called these behaviors "scorching the village." Your village is where you live. Your relationships are important. Don't burn them down, especially now.

It may seem impossible, but you *can* find a healthy outlet for your anger and other emotions, even when you feel like screaming at everyone. Anger and fear are common in grief, but your loved ones may not be able to support you while you're expressing strong emotions. Even if they want to, they may not have the training or skill to manage their own emotions, much less be able to hold steady for yours.

Paul Denniston has developed a very effective mindful movement practice focused on moving these emotions called Grief Yoga.[4] There are other anger-releasing types of exercise that you don't have to study. You can just safely release your anger by hitting or yelling into a pillow. I know it sounds silly,

but try it! Your pillow will never tell you, "I just can't be around you right now. It's too hard."

Another safe way to express emotions is to write them out and witness them yourself. You can learn so much about how you're feeling with a pen and paper! Journaling doesn't have to be a tedious or painful process. Think of it as encouraging movement of stuck energy, removing boulders from your path. You know that relief you feel when nausea churns up your insides for hours and then you finally vomit? Journaling is like that for emotions. Let them out! You'll feel relief.

You can write about anything. There are no rules. Just write. Once, I filled an entire page of a journal with one single word (a four-letter word that starts with f, and it was not "free"), repeated over and over. I used plenty of exclamation points, underlines, and capitals, and I felt a lot of relief after fighting through that page.

Is there a thought that's been bothering you a lot? Sometimes I found it much more helpful to write about a frustration rather than repeat it over and over again to a beloved listening friend, which was better for both of us! Write about it, without any filtering. You don't have to worry about being judged by the page. Just let it out. It doesn't have to make any sense or be in any order; just let the words flow onto the page and see how you feel. Your friends may tire of you saying the same thing repeatedly for months, but your journal never gives you that look like it's heard it all before.

There are endless practices available when it comes to writing. Just write.

I once wrote an entire haiku (a three-line poem with syllabic rules of five/seven/five) using only one single four-letter word. I wrote it five times on the first line, seven times on the second line, and five times again on the third line. It felt good.

Writing can also keep alive your deep, loving connection with your partner. You can write to your loved one. I often talk to or write to Glen and other people who have left my life. It helps me keep them close. What I realized after a while is that even though he's gone, Glen and I still have a relationship. It's different, of course, but I can still love him, think of him, ask him questions, and connect to his guidance.

I keep a journal by my bed. When I'm frustrated and need to process something, I write. Sometimes poems or thoughts for this book come out. Sometimes I just write a string of four-letter words and release anger onto the page. In fact, I've been so deep into releasing I've broken pens before! Sometimes I open the journal to write and then heave it across the room, where it slams against the wall. Any of those actions can be helpful in the moment. You can also tear up or burn the pages after you write, further releasing the emotions you are processing. (Burn them in a fireplace or somewhere safe. Not your bed!)

One day, you may want to look back on your journal as a way of measuring the progress you've made on your journey. Maybe, now that they are written down, you will share your experiences with others in hopes of bringing some meaning to your grief. Looking back, even months from now, you will see that you don't feel exactly the same. Feelings shift and change, and that's okay!

If you don't like to write, try video or audio vlogging, or draw, color, or create with clay or paint. Any way you move your story through you can help soften tension and process your emotions. Start with one sentence, or even a word. Just a minute or two can start moving your story in a healing direction.

The Healing Power of Your Story

At some point, maybe months or years from now, I recommend writing out your story. It doesn't have to be in any way that makes sense or is "readable." It can be just for you to remember and see later how much progress you've made. Writing out my story, with the help of a book coach and the intention to publish it, gave me purpose. Writing helped me sort through and process my experiences and find ways to cope with some of the terrible things that happened. When trauma and grief are locked away, they don't have a path to healing. Shame can only live in secret. Writing can bring all those difficult feelings into the light for processing and even release.

Writing my stories was like bringing a bright light into my grief cave and allowing me to see all of my experiences without judging myself harshly. While I was writing, I would try to frame the stories for someone I was trying to help. This allowed me to see how much shame and guilt I felt and know that not only was that not going to help me, it wasn't going to help anyone else either. I was able to relive, recount, and reframe some of those awful times. I wrote as if I were writing to a trusted friend, which allowed me to judge myself less harshly.

Writing your story can help clarify how you feel about things. It can sort what happened into more manageable pieces, like chapters, so you can find areas that still need processing, identify the pain and where it's coming from, and eventually release more of it. The process can feel similar to being in a good therapist's office, but you can do it in bed at two in the morning. As amazing as my therapist is, she's not available at 2 a.m. Try it. You may find writing soothing. After you've released your feelings onto the page, sit quietly for a moment and breathe; you might be surprised at the ease you find.

I continue to be surprised by how my feelings have evolved since I first started writing my story in 2017. Even though the facts of what actually happened don't change, what does change is our relationship to the story and how it feels. Because of the stories I've written (and talk therapy), I can now talk about most of my experiences from the time around Glen's death without feeling like I need to crawl back into my grief cave and hide. I feel grief, of course. I want things not to have happened the way they did, for sure, but I am empowered by the fact that sharing my story and the practices I use to live a full life helps my healing journey as well as my clients and my readers.

Perceived Fault and Guilt

For a long time after Glen's death, I believed his death was my fault. The note he sent me before he ended his life was full of blame. When people told me it wasn't my fault, I reluctantly agreed because it was easier than arguing. But honestly, I believed I was part of the reason he ended his life. I spent anguished days wondering what I could have done differently to change this horrible outcome, feeling terribly guilty as I replayed the last conversation we had the night before he died, beating myself up and berating myself for not hugging him harder the last time we saw each other. No matter how many times well-meaning friends, and my therapist, reassured me that it wasn't my fault, it didn't help loosen the suffocating choke hold guilt and shame had on me. If I could have accepted my feelings *and* the fact that there was nothing I could have done to change things, I would have started on the path to healing so much earlier. If I could have accepted that I can't change the past, it would have provided some relief. But I spent weeks and months letting regret, shame, and guilt rule.

A full five years after Glen died, during my studies with David Kessler to obtain my grief educator certification, I finally

accepted the past as it was and released myself from the final bit of guilt I had been clinging to.

David told a story about a hospital with a floor specifically designed for suicidal patients. The patient rooms are designed with complete safety in mind. The patients are monitored, and the most highly trained nurses and doctors care for them. Still, suicides happen there. If a place like that can't prevent suicide, how could you, a regular person not trained in suicide prevention, have stopped your partner's suicide? People who die by suicide have issues beyond our ability to help them. My husband was in so much pain that he believed he needed to end his suffering by ending his life. For months, I had tried to convince him not to—to convince him he couldn't leave his kids or me. We tried counseling, yoga, meditation, and medication, but he got worse and worse. I didn't believe it at first, but with lots of time, work, education, and therapy, I now know I couldn't have done anything to prevent his death.

You couldn't stop your partner's suicide, but there are things you *can* control.

A friend of mine says, "Stop shoulding on yourself." Remember, you can't change the past, and the shoulda coulda woulda loops are not helping you. In fact, they are all forms of self-harm, and you are going through enough right now. The last thing you need to do is pick on yourself. Be as kind and gentle with yourself as you would be with a loved one—someone you care deeply about going through the same thing. This is key. All those people telling you it's not your fault—you would do the same, right? Reassure yourself, and do your best to believe it. If there truly had been something you could have done to prevent your partner's death, you would have done it. The fact is, there isn't anything you could have done. And there isn't anything you can do now to change what's happened. You can, however,

change your relationship with what's happened so you don't have to suffer so much.

One tool that might help when you become aware that you're stuck in a story is simply adding the word "and." I learned this tool during my studies with David Kessler. I wish I had had this when I was ruminating about the last conversation I had with Glen. I shoulded on myself more about that one phone call than almost everything else combined. Just once, when I was shoulding about that phone call, if I had added "and" to my rant, it may have shifted my thinking. Try it next time you find yourself repeating something that feels hopeless and painful. My example: "I wish I would have just said yes to seeing me when he called and asked the night before he died, *AND* I couldn't have known it was the night before he died, so I couldn't have acted any differently." When you are ready, this simple tool can give you a big burden release!

I'm not saying it's easy to accept the past, but by accepting it, we can release its pain and, through self-acceptance, let the past guide us to become stronger and more self-sufficient as we create our better future.

"What Do I Do Now?"

Early in our marriage, Glen and I were buried in stress as we tried to build our new life together while merging six children, helping his ex-wife move closer so he and I could live together, fighting a lawsuit with my ex-husband, and dealing with many, many strained relationships with people who thought our marriage was a mistake. We didn't intend to create so much drama, of course. We were just deeply in love and wanted to be together, but our marriage had unexpected ripple effects throughout our lives. More like a tidal wave than a ripple. The number of stressors was overwhelming and caused us a lot of anxiety. Glen was a planner and organizer. He was also great under pressure, so each time we were faced with another stressful turn on our journey, he would say, "This is not the crocodile closest to the canoe." Whatever was at the top of the list of things that needed immediate attention was the crocodile closest to the canoe.

After Glen died, I was so deep in grief, I could only see crocodiles overtaking my canoe. Every challenge looked life-threatening, and I was unable to figure out which one to deal with first. I asked over and over, "What do I do now?"

Use the Notebook to Manage and Track Assets

To help me determine which crocodile I needed to face each day, I had a notebook that I carried everywhere. It had lots of room for papers, including copies of Glen's death certificate, bills, and a handwritten spreadsheet containing all the companies and organizations I needed to contact regarding Glen's death, debts, and all the other details.

Due to grief, trauma, overwhelm, and shock, I was completely incapable of creating something like this at that time. So how did I do it?

Asset Assessment: Helpers are Assets!

While checking your backpack at this rest stop, one thing to keep in mind is that supportive people, with skills you may not have, can also ease your way. Is there a particularly helpful person at your bank or your lawyer's office, or do you have a really organized friend? In my case, I was blessed that my financial advisor was also a compassionate, caring friend who sat with me several times, sifting through the mounds of paperwork and trying to help me figure everything out. He's the one who made the spreadsheet. I still have it, with his neat handwriting and check marks. Sometimes he would leave my house and give me a single task—a single phone call to make or letter to mail. Sometimes even that was too much for me. But when I had a moment of energy, I could refer to that spreadsheet. And like walking through knee-deep mud, I plodded along, and with him cheering me on, I got through it. It took almost two years to finish processing Glen's estate. I want to reassure you, no matter

what condition your partner's assets and debts are in, the estate *will* close. It *will* end.

Make a list in your notebook of the friends, family members, professionals, and people you know who might be able to help you with the tasks that can't wait. During the first few weeks after your partner died, remember how many people said, "Let me know what I can do," and "How can I help?" They're still out there, and there is no time limit on those offers. Even though months may have passed and it seems like everyone has gone back to their lives, they just need a reminder that you're still in need. All the energy they've been storing up to help you is still there, waiting for the ask.

One night, over a year after Glen died, I was trying to make a spreadsheet for estate taxes. I was so frustrated, I was in tears. So I posted on Facebook that if anyone had spreadsheet and accounting abilities, I was in great need of support. Within an hour, a friend of Glen's was at my house, rolling up his sleeves, and he had that job finished in just a few hours. I felt like I'd been blessed with an angel. Don't give up—there is someone out there who can help you! One thing to keep in mind here is that all of this is much, much easier for someone else to manage. Someone who doesn't cry every time they read the death certificate they are about to mail. Someone whose head is clear and whose body isn't telling them a bear is chasing them. It may feel impossible to manage this stuff, and that's because you've just suffered a terrible, traumatizing loss. That backpack is super heavy right now. A trusted friend or accountant can take all the paperwork weight out of the backpack, which will give you a boost on your journey.

Your first task is to reach out when you need it. Believe me, your helpers will be happy to hear from you and happy to help. Supporters of suicide loss survivors feel so helpless—giving them something to do is like giving them a gift. And if they are also

grieving the loss of your partner, a conversation about it will lighten their journey as well.

Checklist of To-Dos

What do you need to do right now? The biggest struggle early on can be figuring out what to do *first*. I struggled with thinking I had to do everything at once, and I didn't prioritize well. So here's a checklist of things that need to be done immediately.

1. Death Certificates

The funeral home may have already helped you with this, but if not, get at least ten copies and be sure at least half of them are the "long form" because some organizations will need that one. It's the one that has the cause of death on it so either prepare yourself or have someone else do the faxing or mailing of this one.

2. Notify

Notifying everyone about your partner's death is a great task to give someone close to you who wants something to do. Try to notify every person, both personal and professional, who knew your partner. You'll be surprised by how many people care and want to know what happened. In fact, you may feel your privacy is invaded by this one, but your partner had relationships with many people, and for their healing to begin, they need to know. You absolutely do not need to provide details, but people will ask. This is another great reason to have someone else do the notifying.

If you can, decide what you do and do not feel comfortable sharing before you begin telling everyone. If people press you for details you are not comfortable sharing, DON'T SHARE. You

are not obligated to provide details. Share what you feel you can. Just keep in mind that when people die, especially by suicide, the shock will cause immediate fear in the people hearing the news, and for them to feel some control over managing their shock, they may ask a lot of questions. They aren't trying to be rude; they are simply trying to manage their feelings.

3. Create a Grieving Space

People need to grieve. As the partner, you are the primary mourner, and therefore everyone will look to you for guidance about grieving. If you have a funeral or a memorial, great; everyone can come and share their condolences. If you aren't up to having a service, start a page on Facebook or another app where people can gather virtually to tell stories and share their grief. Better yet, have a friend do this for you. If you are short on funds, ask someone to start a GoFundMe or other crowdfunding group where people can not only share their grief but also donate to support you.

4. Start the Tasks

In your notebook, make a clear checklist of tasks, even if the first and only one you are up to writing right now is "make a task list." If you can create a list, you will feel a tiny bit of control returning to your life, and this will ease your suffering.

Here is a list of organizations you'll need to contact. Some will need death certificates to close accounts. Always ask if a copy of the death certificate is sufficient and save the originals for when necessary, since there is a cost to order more.

- your partner's employer

- clubs, gyms, and any other activities
  that may have a membership

- credit cards (some of them might allow you to
  delay payment until the estate is closed)

- subscriptions (if you can't find these, refer to a
  credit card statement or bank statement)

- look for charges from utility companies, phone bills, and
  anything that might need to be paid immediately, and
  contact the company asking for an extension if needed

- bank

- health insurance

- estate attorney (Hopefully, your partner had a will. If not,
  you'll still need an attorney to manage assets and make sure
  the estate is distributed according to your state's laws.)

Of course, this is not a complete list, and whether or not you were married will have a big impact on how the estate is processed. But this is a good start. If you have an estate attorney, they will provide all the details you need. If you have a friend who lost a partner or spouse, they will be able to guide you. You don't need to reinvent the wheel here; use others' experience.

Make a spreadsheet with a column for each organization you have contacted, the date you contacted them, the method (email, phone number, etc.), and what further action, if any, is required. Things like utilities, shared bank accounts, etc., will require a death certificate to remove your spouse's name and have it put in your name only.

I know this sounds like a lot, but if you just take one small step when you are able, you'll get through it.

Get as much help as possible.

Tap your friends who are great at spreadsheets, managing banks and other financial institutions, health insurance and hospital bills, and any other crocodiles circling your canoe. The burden will feel much lighter if you spread the tasks among your supporters.

Small Goals

Days after Glen died, when the medical examiner had released his body, I had to go to the funeral home. My friend was waiting to drive me there because I was in no shape to drive—I was shaking most of the time and could hardly focus on a task for a minute, much less the fifteen minutes it would take to drive there. I was in my closet trying to get dressed. On a normal day, I could do this activity without thinking, but still in shock, I had to literally coach myself through every step. I had to name and choose one item of clothing at a time. I stood in my closet wondering what order the clothes should go on my body; I had to really think hard about it. It took overwhelming focus and energy to do a simple daily task that normally would take little thought and effort. Everything was so difficult! It was like only part of me was there, and it wasn't the part that knew how to get dressed.

One simple task is too much? Break it down into micro tasks: one sock at a time, one shoe at a time, one breath at a time.

Memorializing

Glen talked about his death a lot and made his wishes very clear to me from the beginning of our relationship. At first, I was resistant to even listening. I would tell him, "Can you *not* be planning your memorial now, when we've just met and married?" Even though it upset me, I got used to his macabre sense of humor—constantly threatening to haunt me to be sure I was having a fun life after he died. Eventually, and with the help of my therapist, I came to accept that death is just a reality in the minds of certain people. I believe talking about and planning for what happened after his death was just a way for him to feel in control.

He repeatedly told me that he wanted his ashes spread in a place where we had great joy. "I don't want a funeral. I just want you and our friends to get together and have a giant party. No viewing, no burial, no graveside, just torch me up and spread my ashes somewhere beautiful." He wanted his ashes taken on a jump with his Navy SEAL brothers and had emphasized, "I do not want a military burial. I do not want to be in a military cemetery, and absolutely no way do I want anyone to ever hand you a flag."

All these conversations and proclamations Glen had made throughout our relationship were ringing in my ears in the days following his death and generating so many conflicting thoughts and feelings. I was beyond stressed out and confused. And with trauma and grief squeezing my brain, I could barely make a decision about what to eat or wear or do, much less big decisions like how to properly memorialize him. I wanted to honor his wishes, but I was also under pressure from his family. His closest aunt wanted a viewing and was going to fly all the way from the East Coast for that.

I wanted to support everyone's wishes, and I was terrified I would do the wrong thing. While desperately searching for the "right" thing to do in the face of all the conflicting needs and desires from everyone who loved and cared about Glen, something my mother said while she was battling cancer just nine years earlier came to mind. I could hear her voice as clearly as if she were standing right next to me. During her three-and-a-half-year battle with leukemia, she wouldn't commit to anything having to do with her memorial because she wanted to make sure we, as her family members, were getting our desires met. "Life is for the living, Michelle. Once someone is gone, you need to take care of those who are left behind."

I wrestled with the right thing to do even as one of our friends, two days after Glen's death, asked if I wanted to donate Glen's brain to research on traumatic brain injury (TBI) and PTSD. That question knocked me over.

I'm guessing you've experienced some feelings like this, especially just after your loved one died. In retrospect, if I could have helped others by donating Glen's brain, I would have done it. But at the time, I couldn't even comprehend that he was dead, much less think about donating his brain.

How can you plan a memorial for someone when you can't even believe they're dead? I agonized over the decision. Finally, I decided to plan a memorial that allowed the people who knew and loved him to grieve while also connecting with what would be meaningful for me.

I had the funeral home prepare his body for a viewing so his aunt and his kids could see him. I was raised Jewish, and it was so far from any tradition I was comfortable with, so I didn't even consider viewing his body because, of course, I had already seen it. After the viewing for his aunt, I had his body cremated, per his request. His ashes were divided between his kids, his family,

other loved ones who requested them, and some were delivered to his SEAL buddies. When I went to the funeral home to pick up his ashes, they handed me a flag. "We know your husband served in the military, and we want to thank you for his service." I held that flag and cried for hours and told Glen I was sorry that this wish of his had been negated.

Two weeks after his death, on a sunny afternoon, all of his local friends and family gathered in a large hall where I held a memorial service. My daughter and her friend sang; his daughter read a poem; and work colleagues and friends spoke. Two of his military buddies did a flag ceremony and handed the flag to Glen's son. After the service, we ate some of Glen's favorite foods and sat and told stories about him. "Life is for the living." I could hear my mom's words supporting me throughout this terrible event. I gave the living a chance to grieve in community, and it felt as right as anything could at that time.

Jewish tradition guides us to gather and say prayers daily for a week after a death. I didn't have a traditional shiva, but after Glen's memorial, I invited my Jewish community to my home for a minyan (a gathering of ten or more Jewish people) and to say kaddish (a prayer recited while memorializing). I've always thought it interesting that we say a prayer that doesn't actually talk about death after someone dies, but I believe it's a supportive prayer to remind us that life is for the living, and even in the worst of times, we always have God to be grateful for.

A few months after his death, Glen's son asked to spread his portion of the ashes in a place where the two of them had a joyful time together. Listening to his son comment on the texture of the ashes as he dropped them from high in a tree over our favorite lake and then jump into the water as he had done with his father before was poignant and heart-wrenching. But

something about it felt good; I could almost feel Glen smiling and laughing with his son.

Sometimes memorials don't go as expected.

I spread some of his ashes in Maui, Hawaii with a friend and my daughter that same summer, but I remember feeling nothing. It was the strangest feeling. My daughter had created a plumeria lei, as Hawaiian tradition suggests. I'd paddled out into the ocean with my friend who also loved Glen, where we laid the lei on the water and poured the ashes through the circle. My friend said a few words about Glen and how their bond was formed and had felt, but I could find no words, nor could I feel anything. I just sat on my paddleboard, frozen, staring at the water, watching his ashes dissipate into the blue. Even though I knew this was what he wanted, I didn't feel a connection to Glen or his joy.

A year to the day after he died, I was back in Maui with the rest of his ashes and went alone to a beach which was the site of, in Glen's words, the most heroic act of his life. He loved telling this story about how, while we were snorkeling in murky, churned-up water, he had saved me from a turtle that was trying to kill me. I could see the smile on his face and hear his laughter. I was so connected to him that day as I poured his ashes into the ocean. I even had a visit from a turtle! I felt pure love for Glen and admiration for all he tried to do in this world. I felt sorrow for losing him and compassion for his pain. This was my own private memorial, and I felt deeply connected to him. At that moment, I was fully grieving, and the tears flowed.

Those were the big memorials, but there continue to be countless smaller ones. Anything that honors his life is a memorial. When I drank the last cup of the coffee he had bought me from my favorite bean roaster, I thought of him with gratitude.

For years, on the anniversary of his death, I visited the spot where I found his body. I lit a candle or put down flowers, sat,

breathed, and focused completely on him. I know he would think that was silly and that I should have been memorializing him by having fun doing something crazy or outrageous, but for some reason, that felt right. The last time I visited the place where he died, I could feel it was the final time. A concrete parking lot was not where he was dwelling; I no longer felt close to him there, and I never went back. Now on the anniversary of his death, I do something he would have loved, like watch *Mars Attacks* (his favorite terrible movie) or eat a donut (nutrition, forgive me).

Another Jewish tradition is observing the anniversary of a loved one's death, their yahrzeit. It is said that a person has two deaths—the day their body dies and the day their name is spoken for the last time. Weekly, at our Friday night and Saturday morning services, the names of people whose yahrzeits fall that week are read out loud. Even though Glen was not Jewish, my rabbi reads his name every year on that anniversary, keeping his memory alive.

When I see his children and I see that twinkle in their eye, just like their father's, I think of him. Each mindful moment I bring his memory into my heart, take a deep breath, and sometimes even speak to him, I memorialize him.

No doubt you have given the idea of memorializing some thought. Just remember, you did not do it wrong. There are many ways to memorialize, and just like grieving, it doesn't matter how long it's been since the death or how you do it—if it is meaningful for you, you're doing it right.

Their Stuff

Have you been asking yourself, "What do I do with all of their stuff?" Stuff is tough.

Another big burden that needs to be released to lighten your journey is your partner's stuff. Do you look around at their things and feel overwhelmed? How are you possibly going to manage getting it to all the "right" places? Or maybe the day they died, you threw away everything they owned. Either way, even if you've already gotten rid of most everything, what remains of their stuff may be weighing you down. Again, just like grief, there is nothing you can do here that is wrong.

One thing I do recommend is to not make any quick decisions. If you can't stand the sight of something right now, you may feel differently later. So for now, unburden yourself by getting rid of what you are sure will never feel important or sentimental to you and keep everything else. If it hurts you to look at these things—if you want all their stuff out of the house but don't want to get rid of it yet—then move it into storage or simply pack it into boxes and hide them in the back of a closet or another room. Don't have room to store them? Remember those helpful people I keep mentioning? If any of them have a spare room or space in their garage or storage unit, they may be happy to house the stuff until you can go through it when it's less painful. It will get easier!

It's so easy to get caught up in uncertainty when it comes to your partner's stuff. Of course, their family may want some of their things, but if you aren't ready to part with things, you are allowed to say, "Please wait. I'm not ready!" Whether you put things in storage or leave them exactly where they are, you'll have them when you are ready to figure out what to do with them.

If you can't make a decision about something, don't. There is no rush. The people who want and need these things will be there when you're ready to part with them. You may find that after your spouse died, you felt connected to an organization that supported you through this time, and you may want to donate to them so they can repurpose or reuse some things.

There is no wrong choice here. Whatever your heart tells you to do is right.

Mindfulness can help with this as well. Spend a moment with each item you're trying to make a decision about. Close your eyes and breathe deeply into your belly. See if you can connect with how you feel about the item. Guidance from this practice may be a clear, "get rid of it," or "give it to _____," or "keep it," or you may not get any answer. Don't rush. Keep trying. The answer will come to you when the time is right.

If you aren't ready to let go of that smelly T-shirt, then don't. Some things may be out of your control, like when you need to return to work. But with the things you can control, like when to wash that T-shirt that still smells like him, you're in charge. If someone tells you differently, it's likely because they're uncomfortable with that dirty T-shirt being around, and that's their problem, not yours. Hang on to that smelly thing until you're ready to wash it. That's true of any of their stuff. If it brings you joy, or some sort of connection with them, hang on to it for as long as it feels right. If you aren't sure, keep it and decide later, because once it's gone, it's gone. Hang on until you feel more

sure. Eventually, with mindful practice, the decisions about what to do with stuff will come easier.

Memorializing Their Stuff

As I mentioned earlier, I did end up with an American flag, and at first, I felt terrible about it. Just looking at it gave me all these terrible feelings, knowing Glen didn't want me to have one. Having absolutely no idea what to do with it, and being unable to look at it, I threw it into the back of my closet. The trouble was that whenever I was looking for that lost sweatshirt or handbag, I came across the protective bag from the funeral home that said "Dignity," and it sent me into a grieving moment all over again. It kept surprising me, terribly.

Eventually, I moved it to the back of the cabinet where I keep cleaning supplies and cat food. This felt very disrespectful, but at least I couldn't keep accidentally running into it in my closet. Years passed, and I still couldn't figure out what to do with the flag. I was also feeling a lot of guilt because I have respect for the flag, for our armed forces, and for what Glen's service to our country meant, but I felt I was disrespecting all of that by hiding the flag in the back of a cabinet because I couldn't bear to look at it. I asked my neighbor, who served in the Navy for forty-plus years, for his suggestion, and he told me the story of his father's flag. He told me how proud he was to hang the full-size flag every holiday. I began to feel a strong urge to do something with my flag, but I was so conflicted, I couldn't make a choice. When I asked my therapist, I was given the same advice I gave you in the previous section: "When the time is right, you will know what to do with it."

And then, just like my therapist said, one Memorial Day five years after Glen died, I was able to take out the flag. I looked at it, held it, and thought about all it represented. It didn't feel terrible like it had every other time I had looked at it. I was able to touch it lovingly and imagine Glen being annoyed but supportive. I may have yelled something like, "Well, you idiot, if you would have stayed here, you could have told me more stories about what you didn't want done with this flag." (By the way, did I mention it's okay to talk to your spouse/partner? And did I also mention you can say anything and everything you want? It's a great way to process feelings. You're doing it for your health. Just maybe not out loud in the middle of the street or in a crowded area—you might get some funny looks. I know, because I have actually done this.)

I googled "what to do with a memorial flag" and researched all the many possibilities. Finally, I decided to get a personalized flag memorial box and ordered one from Etsy.com. I requested the glass be etched with his name, the dates of his birth and death, and "Proud Frog Man, I Will Not Fail.," a Navy SEAL credo. I added a trident pin, although it didn't fit in the flag case, so now it rests next to the flag in a place of pride on the shelf in my family room.

There are also artistic and fun ways to memorialize stuff. You can make (or have made) a stuffed animal or pillow out of their favorite shirt, or frame it and put it on the wall with notes and cards arranged artfully around it. You can make a quilt or blanket out of photos of them. Check out Pinterest.com or Etsy.com for more ideas on how to preserve your loved one's stuff. There is no wrong here. Do what makes you feel good.

Another "stuff management challenge" that I faced was what to do with our wedding rings. I fretted and sweated and left them in a box in my nightstand drawer for years until the right

idea came to me. I purchased a small ornate box with a design of Celtic knots, a nod to Glen's Irish heritage. The rings are stored on the same shelf next to the beautiful flag case. Finally, after all those years, the memorializing of those most important items is complete. I know it's complete because when I placed those items on the "altar," I felt lighter. And when I look at them, I know they are part of my world—reminders of difficult but also beautiful experiences and the precious life of my love.

When you are unburdening yourself of your partner's stuff, aim for that feeling, and if you can't get even close, then maybe it's not time. I was almost at the six-year mark when that memorial shelf was complete. You may be at one year or forty years, but when you are calm and connected to your body and remembering the love you two shared, you will know what's right. You'll know because your heart will tell you.

People Unable to Support You

I lost my mom to cancer when she was seventy and I was forty-one. At the time, it was the most traumatic experience of my life. In fact, I remember telling myself then that nothing would ever hurt as much as that loss. As difficult as it was, I did learn some very important lessons about loss, grief, and people. Those lessons helped some when Glen died, but of course, I had so much more to learn.

You may have already experienced this, or possibly you are experiencing this, and you just don't realize it because you already feel so awful, but not everyone is able to support you while you're grieving. In fact, some of those who are hovering around you right now to "support" you may actually be adding weight to your backpack and obstacles to your journey. It doesn't make sense, right? Just when you need people to be their strongest and most supportive, they are failing to make you feel better and aren't able to take care of your needs. Understanding why this happens can be helpful in easing the extra burden of those relationships.

Bring to mind the image of a tornado. When your partner dies by suicide, it can feel like a tornado blew in and destroyed your world. As the spouse or partner, you are in the center of

the destructive path of this tornado. The destruction, however, was beyond your house; your "neighborhood" was also damaged. This includes all the family and friends who are also mourning. There are people who you may not even know had a relationship with your partner, who seemed like a distant acquaintance, but are nonetheless grieving and suffering because of your spouse's death. If you can think of it this way, you may have an easier time understanding that not everyone you usually rely upon for support will be able to help you now. They may be unable to withstand even a tiny wind, so they may retreat for safety.

This can be very frustrating and disappointing, but the fact is suicide loss is an incredibly difficult thing to be strong around. Instead of helping you, they need support themselves because they're too overwhelmed by their own shock and grief to be there for you. This is why it is necessary to get a nonjudgmental, uninvolved third party, specifically a therapist, counselor, or coach with specialized training in grief. Believe it or not, many people with degrees in mental health have had little or no training in grief, so choose wisely.

I just want to take a moment here and say I'm sorry. I'm sorry that you're suffering from this terrible, traumatic experience. And I'm sorry some of the people around you may be disappointing, adding weight to your backpack and obstacles to your journey instead of helping. I'm sorry all your needs may not be getting taken care of by the people you want to rely on.

They Are Suffering Too

If you can maintain an awareness of people's limitations, you will feel less resentful and let down.

When Glen died, I had a very close friend who was a mental health crisis counselor. He worked in a hospital with the severely mentally ill. Because of this special training, I thought he would be the best support when everyone around me seemed unable to cope, much less support me. At first, my friend was a great help; he checked in at least by phone almost daily and visited often. Then a few months after Glen died, I noticed my friend had stopped contacting me. It devastated me. I trusted him and had begun to rely on our frequent talks for his wisdom and support. When he finally came to visit after a few weeks of absence, he complimented me on how strong I was. I was so tired of hearing that! (Raise your hand if you're tired of being told how strong you are!) Then he told me he was struggling with suicidal thoughts and that he couldn't be around me. I tried to be supportive, but with so little in my tank, I really couldn't help him. He left my life for months after that, compounding my loss. I was devastated to lose one of my few professionally qualified supporters, but now I know he was hurting too, and he couldn't take care of himself, much less lend support to me. Instead of being mad at him and disappointed in our troubled friendship, which added weight to my backpack, I could more easily have accepted that we just couldn't be there for each other at that time. I could have reassured myself that this was all temporary and that we could be friends again someday when we weren't both in crisis.

Many months later, we reconnected. He was in a terrible state, but I was stronger and more able to be the friend he needed. That is, until he threatened his own suicide. He explained how he had it all planned and told me, a few days later on the phone, that he was going to do it that evening. This was a huge trauma activator for me. I took him seriously and did what I regret never doing with Glen. I took a deep breath and called the suicide hotline. I knew I couldn't personally help him, and this crisis needed to

be managed by people trained to do so. I wasn't helpless, and I wanted to do what I could. My friend was furious with me, at first, because the authorities came to his workplace. Eventually, he forgave me and understood the terrible position I had been in. When Glen started threatening suicide, I never believed him. He also told me he would never go if the police came to take him to the hospital. I figured that was true, so I didn't call. Now in the same situation, I didn't hesitate to make the call to get my friend the professional help he needed. To have done what I didn't do for Glen eased some of the guilt I was feeling.

It may feel unfair, and it would be just perfect if everyone who wasn't the partner, the primary mourner, could put their own crap aside and just be there for you. But like you, they are human and have also experienced this loss in their own way. Those people you wish could be supporting you have backgrounds and experiences that cause their grief to be different from yours. Try not to judge others for how they are grieving and absolutely don't let anyone judge you!

Some days, it may seem like even your supportive friend is more upset than you are, and that might feel frustrating or confusing. It will help you if you can remember that everyone around you who is trying to help and be supportive have big challenges to overcome that make it difficult to impossible for them to be there for you.

They Are Grieving Too

They are dealing with their own feelings of loss, fear, grief, and sorrow about your partner's suicide. They have their own version of a grief cave to hide in and a healing journey to regain their lives. Their mountain may not be as steep and their backpack lighter,

but they still need to endure their own climb. Even though you are the primary mourner, people who may not have been that close to your partner are still grieving, going through a process that may or may not mirror or coordinate with yours. If you can keep that in mind, it will help you when you feel frustrated or disappointed by some "support" that is not supportive.

I ran into this almost immediately when one of my friends came over to "comfort" me the day after Glen died. She expressed her pain as anger and spent the whole time asking me probing questions about the state I found Glen's body in, our last conversation, and other insensitive questions that traumatized me further. She also fretted loudly about how horrible Glen was for doing this to us; she called him a coward and selfish. Her behavior upset me so much that I stepped out of my usual "take care of everyone" mode and asked her husband to take her home and not bring her back. When I saw her again weeks later, we talked it out. I explained that I knew she was hurting, but I could not be around her pain because it made me feel worse. She was processing her own grief and needed to get help elsewhere. Setting boundaries was one of my weakest relationship skills, and this was the beginning of my growth in that area.

If you are experiencing this with your friends, try on a phrase like:

"I love you, but right now, I cannot have this conversation. I need a break from it."

"When you express your anger, I feel more upset and have to manage my feelings and yours. Let's take a break."

While I was learning to do this, I took a rest-and-assess break to determine who would be the best person to call to take over my backpack for this section of the journey. I figured out who that might be and called and said, "I just need you to confirm to me that Glen was not a selfish, weak asshole..." and my friend did that and more. She helped me remember what a loving, giving, joyful person he was; she reminded me how he loved me so deeply; and she listened while I told stories about him. That's what I needed at that moment. Another time, I may have needed to release anger and frustration and call him names, and then I would call the friend who was right for that. Choosing the right support for what you need in the moment will lighten your backpack and fuel you.

You are not responsible for their suffering.
Stay in your lane.

Sometimes during the grief journey, paths can merge and cross and even get mixed up. Most of the people coming in and out of your daily life right now likely have some feelings about your partner's death. As I've mentioned, your journey is yours alone. This doesn't mean you are alone—you are never alone because you have supporters, friends and family, and therapists and coaches who can share the burden and be with you. Your journey is yours because no one else has the experience you are having. Everyone affected by the loss of your partner must go through a healing journey of their own. They can't do the grieving work for you any more than you can do the grieving work for them. It gets confusing, especially if you have children or siblings who were closely involved in your relationship with your partner.

David Kessler taught me this analogy, and it has helped me and my clients tremendously when our grief gets mixed up with others' grief.

Think of your journey as a trip down a freeway. Each person grieving the loss of your partner is in their own car. Each lane is individual, and there is only one car per lane.

You need to stay in your lane, driving at the speed that feels comfortable for you and stopping to gather support for your journey as you need.

Your supporters and everyone else on the freeway with you must also stay in their lanes. Lane crossing, as you can imagine, only ends in chaos and a more difficult journey.

An example: Your partner's sister is having a very challenging journey. She has the equivalent of a flat tire, but she has roadside assistance in the form of her own supporters. You need all your resources and likely do not have an extra tire for her. When she's up and running again, you can meet at a rest stop to support each other, but you are not responsible for getting her there. Of course, if you do feel like you can spare a tire (and you may sometimes feel fueled up and strong), then by all means, assist her!

Team Up and Get Help

Another thing to keep in mind is that unless you are lucky enough to have someone educated in grief around, the people in your support system usually don't know what to do. In our culture, we do not have in-depth training or even open communication about how to process and integrate the grief experience. Nor are we educated about how to support grievers, especially when the loss has a social stigma attached to it, like suicide does. When those friends say, "Let me know what you need!" or "Let me know what I can do for you," they really don't know, and they really are asking. They need direction, advice, and guidance on how best to support you. Which sucks, because wouldn't it be

nice if they would just take care of your needs without you having to coordinate it all?

Think about what would lighten your backpack right now. Who is the right person to walk beside you and carry some of the load during this next part of your journey?

About a week after Glen died, I had two friends helping me organize things. One set up a fund to cover my bills and to help Glen's ex-wife and kids with their expenses. The other drove me to the funeral home, made sure I had food organized, and picked out a suit for Glen's viewing. Partway through that awful first week, I was walking around lost and destroyed, and someone came over to drop off some food. I looked at my funeral home friend and said, "I should be bringing food to people. I'm not the one who needs care—I'm the one who brings soup and flowers and helps!"

"Michelle," she said to me sincerely, "you are always taking care of others. Your support bank account is full. It's time for you to make a withdrawal." I was deeply grateful for her words; they helped me release the guilt and allowed me to receive and realize that I could lean on these people who were asking what they could do. People were bringing food (way more than I could eat), but they didn't know what else to do. So we sat down and made a list of everything that needed doing, and she matched up people to the tasks. People were very happy to be given an assignment; having a concrete way to help made them feel useful and helped them with their grief.

And if it's been months or even years since your partner died, you can still ask people for help. Go back through your texts or messages on your socials and see how many people in those first few days offered help. There is no expiration date on those offers; people just need to be asked.

There are also support groups online, all over the world. If your loved ones aren't able to be helpful enough, find some

support in your local community or online. There are some great support groups for suicide loss survivors on Grief.com and on social media. People in these groups will understand what you're going through. Be careful, of course. If the group doesn't feel supportive, if you feel worse after having visited it, then get out of there! There is also the 988 Suicide & Crisis Lifeline; you can dial 988 for immediate help. Please consider finding yourself a therapist or a counselor. Having someone in your corner who is not also grieving the person you've lost is so helpful. Their backpack is empty, and it is their sole purpose (and probably soul purpose) to be there to help lighten your load.

Again, you have to be thoughtful when choosing your therapist. Therapy can be very difficult, and there will likely be times when you're very uncomfortable and will want to skip your session because it's just too hard. Please trust that the work you are doing in therapy will set you up for a smoother journey through grief and allow you to grow in the ways you need for healing. It's difficult, but the right therapist will give you the tools you need and help you build strength and resilience for your climb. Sometimes, however, a therapist can be a poor match for you. For example, say it's been eight months since your partner died. You finally feel ready to attempt the climb out of your grief cave and begin your healing journey. You meet your therapist and they say, "Well, by eight months, you should be feeling this way because the pain of grief only really lasts six weeks." (This actually happened to a friend of mine.) Leave. Find a therapist or coach who is trained in grief. It may take a couple of sessions, but some really well-trained professionals are out there, so be patient. You wouldn't hire a mountain climbing guide who wasn't trained and didn't know the terrain, right? This may be the most important helper on your journey, so please choose wisely.

How to Choose a Therapist

Here's a quick guide for finding a therapist to help guide you toward healing:

1. Check with your insurance company and ask what type of therapist (MS, PhD, MD, LPC) is covered and for what length of time or number of visits. If you have no coverage, they may be able to direct you to a local agency that provides therapy.

2. Look through the list and find someone with whom you believe you will resonate. Ask yourself these questions:

    - Do you appreciate the energy of a younger therapist or the calm wisdom of a more experienced one?

    - Are you more comfortable with a specific gender?

    - If you are doing in-person sessions, will the commute be doable?

3. Then find out these things:

    - Are they taking new clients?

    - Do they have grief focus or training in their bio? If not, when you make first contact, ask them if they work with clients in grief. Special training in grief and trauma would be even better.

Once you have chosen a therapist, make sure that you communicate well. This is absolutely key. They need to understand you and your pain, and you need to understand their counseling. Give the therapist a visit or two before you decide if you resonate. This may be a long-term relationship and one of your most important supports for healing.

Therapy is difficult, especially when you are recovering from trauma and in grief. Be patient. You may be really uncomfortable in your therapist's office. Try to determine whether this discomfort is because of the work you're doing to find healing or if the therapist isn't the right one for you. Using mindfulness tools can help. It's hard work, but you will get there. It is possible to journey toward healing and to feel good again.

If your spouse or partner was a military veteran, like Glen was, there are a lot of ways to get support from the military as a survivor. Tragedy Assistance Program for Survivors, TAPS, is a wonderful group. They include survivors no matter what your relationship was or whether they were retired, active duty, or only served a few months. Partner, ex-partner, friend, family—anyone who grieves someone who served is welcome. After TAPS helped me far enough through my grief journey, I became a peer mentor, and that connection continues to nourish me and help me grow as I support other suicide widows.

Find Your People

Here's a tip on how to decide if this is the time to have more or less of a particular person in your life while you are on this journey: use mindfulness! Focus on how you feel when you're about to see this person. Ask yourself if you're looking forward to seeing them or anxious about seeing them. Notice how you feel while you spend time with them and afterward. It's as simple as that. If you feel worse during a visit with them, try to spend less time with them; if you feel better, spend more. If you ask for support and end up feeling more stuck, heavier, drained, betrayed, or more lost, find a different guide. Make your healing your top priority. The more progress you can make on

your healing journey, the more you'll be able to help and support others. That means surrounding yourself with people who can lighten your backpack, show you a smoother, flatter route, and even carry some of the weight for you.

PART 3
THE CLIMB

Building Resilience

I'd love for you to take a minute right now just to check in with yourself. If you're reading this book in order, you've read and taken in a lot of information and hopefully started one or more of the practices. Stop and take a deep breath and just check in: What do you need right now, at this moment? Is it to continue reading, or is it to take a walk, eat some nourishing food, or call a friend? Checking in with yourself and assessing what you need is a practice you'll need to do over and over during your journey. This "listening to your body" skill is one that will help you build resilience as you begin the climb. Resting when you need rest, nourishing yourself when you need fuel, and using calming techniques when you are activated will help ease your way.

It may feel like your climb started the day your loved one died, or possibly even before that, if you were having difficulties, like Glen and I were. But the climb I am referring to here is that of moving along your grief journey with *awareness*. Parts 1 and 2 have helped you develop the invaluable practice of awareness of your feelings, how to calm yourself, and how to release the burdens to make your journey toward healing as light as possible.

As you progress, additional obstacles may make your journey difficult. You may feel like you're off your path or even moving backward sometimes. These obstacles could be anniversaries, a return to work, a complication in the estate, financial hardship, or additional losses. It could be absolutely nothing you're aware of that sends you off your path and into a dark place. That's okay. That's what the grief journey is like. You have the tools of mindfulness, so you know how to be resilient when these dark and difficult times show up. Don't add to the weight by being hard on yourself.

Even when you're doing everything right to take care of yourself, you may have an emotional setback, for known or unknown reasons, and just feel like crap. Try not to add crap

to crap! There are tougher days and easier days; that's how grief works. When you are having the easier days, mindfully recognize them and try to remember, even celebrate them. When you realize you're having a challenging day, practice self-care by phoning a supportive friend, taking a walk, or looking through the exercises in this book and trying one again. Or maybe this is a lie-in-bed-and-just-cry day. Recognizing what you need, and taking care of that need, will lighten your burden. Be gentle with yourself. I used this written list of things I could do because when I was really down, I couldn't immediately think of anything other than picking on myself for being down.

Helpful To-Do List:

- phone a friend
- go for a walk
- eat a favorite food
- watch a beloved movie that gives good feels
- binge an old favorite series, or a new one
- mindfully sip a favorite beverage
- sit outside and connect with nature
- listen to uplifting music or a podcast
- spend time being fully present with a pet
- rub feet with oil
- lie in bed and stare at the ceiling or cry, or both
- shower
- indulge in massage, acupuncture, reiki, chiropractic, other healing modalities

- get out coloring books and crayons
  or colored pencils and color

- draw

- play a board game or card game

- get your journal and write

You will feel better after using the practices I've listed so far, but allow yourself the space to sidestep the path (or fall off the path) and just be with the pain sometimes. Hold yourself in love, along with your pain.

As I have mentioned previously, if any of the practices in this book do not feel supportive or helpful, skip them. Each one will become useful when you're ready and able to take advantage of them. If you can only lie in bed and cry today, do that. Tomorrow, or next week, or next month, you can come back to the book and find support to continue your journey.

Missteps, sidesteps, and obstacles are not insurmountable. When you put the practices of this section into use, you will find a gentle staircase where there was once a steep, rocky path. These staircases, carved into your journey by your strength, will help you build more resilience and ease your way.

STAIRCASE 1

Forgiveness and Prayers

There is a well-known indigenous story about an elder who was teaching a young man about the mind. The elder told the young man, "You have two wolves at war inside you—the wolf of love, joy, and freedom and the wolf of anger, hatred, and violence." The young student asked, "How do we know which wolf will win the war?" The elder replied, "The one you feed."

Forgiveness is the highest form of self-care and a powerful boost for healing. The way to forgiveness is not easy, but once you traverse the terrain, you will gain one of the most powerful wellness tools available. Forgiveness shines a light into the deepest darkness of grief and sorrow. You've heard the saying "Holding a grudge is like drinking poison and waiting for the other person to die." Drinking poison doesn't help us get to where we want to go.

How to Forgive Your Partner

The first step is to remember all the things you consider good about you or your partner, or whomever you are working on forgiving at this time. And work it is! But it's worth every effort. This is feeding the wolf of love. No one is all good or all bad. You may hate your partner right now, but it's worth exploring

how you also loved them and how, way down deep, the love is still there. Right now, it may seem impossible to ever have good feelings about your partner again, but that is the fear of the bear talking. Anger, hatred, frustration—all these feelings are happening because you don't want what happened to have happened. Anger can protect you from grief and sorrow because it's a more empowering emotion. But ultimately, you'll want to feel joy again, to feel lighter and live an enjoyable life. With forgiveness, you can.

It's okay to feel joy, not just heartbreak, when you think of your partner. When you are ready, allow yourself to think of the wonderful, beautiful things your partner brought into your life. There were qualities that attracted you to them and made you feel joy and love. Remember the times when being in their presence boosted your mood and made you feel happy? That love is still there. In fact, the pain you're feeling because of your loss is because of the depth of your love. Focus your awareness and attention on those beautiful moments; grow them and use them as the light in your life, and the darkness will shrink.

With some effort, the day will come when you can greet yourself and your partner with forgiveness and compassion for your suffering and theirs. That pain will ease, and the love can rise to the surface and be the strongest memory. It takes time. You'll know when you are ready, and when you are, take baby steps; some smiles will start to shine through the tears, some memories will begin to be less tainted with bitterness and sorrow. When that happens, notice it, embrace it, and amplify it; focus mindfully on those times!

Ceremony

In Judaism, we perform a ceremony at the New Year—we take bread crumbs, which represent our burdens, misdeeds, guilt, or

anything we need to let go, and release them into a moving body of water. My counselor suggested I write a list or a story that included some of my most difficult and uncomfortable feelings and then burn the paper and set the ashes on the wind. At first, I thought this was silly, but once I tried it, I realized it really did release something. You can throw rocks into water, blow dandelion seeds into the wind, or whatever might be a meaningful action for you. It might take more than one ceremony and some time, but if you set the intention and keep releasing yourself from guilt and your partner from blame, you'll progress.

Mindful Transformation of Emotion

It's also essential to move the old energy out of the body. Remember, emotions are energy in motion and need to be released. For example, if you're overcome with anger and you pick up one of your partner's possessions or a gift from them, and you hurl it against the wall, you *will* get a quick release of anger, but my guess is you won't feel better in the long run, especially if you broke the item. Next time you feel this urge, be angry, but express it by jogging outside, or hitting a pillow, or yelling and screaming (maybe into a pillow so you don't scare anyone). Then, once that energy has moved through you, find a long, slow deep breath; perhaps try one of the breathing techniques I mentioned and begin to calm yourself. When you feel ready, take the object you were about to destroy and hold it as you would your lover's hand when things were good. Look at it, and mindfully use all your senses to be present with it, and instead of focusing on the pain, remember the joy you felt when it came into your life. Things were good then. Feel the love that was part of that time and breathe into it. See if you can pull that feeling out of your memory and surround yourself with it energetically, like a hug. Keep breathing deeply, and see if that object can now transform

into an object that brings you joy. Check in with yourself and see if this practice helped you feel better.

Self-Forgiveness

Forgive yourself for whatever you can. Are you holding on to that last conversation you had? Sometimes I still feel uncomfortable feelings of guilt and shame when I think about the final conversation I had with Glen the night before he died. I accept those feelings and work with them by breathing, and this is where self-forgiveness becomes the only way through the powerful obstacles of shame and guilt. If I continued the self-loathing, guilt, and shame that I felt for what I said during that last conversation, wishing I could change it, I would still be miserable, feeding the wolf of self-loathing. I can't change that last conversation. But with forgiveness practice, I changed how I felt about it and lessened the horror of the memory of it. Now I can remember that conversation and tell myself, "I was doing my best. I had no way of knowing that would be our last conversation." Of course we didn't know that was going to be our last conversation; if we had, we would have done things differently. We did not have the foresight to know when our loved one was going to die, but we have something much more powerful—the power to forgive ourselves for what we didn't know and for our actions because we didn't know.

How do we forgive ourselves? We are so conditioned toward shame, self-loathing, and guilt. I started by working on releasing shame. I reminded myself that I didn't know what was going to happen—I didn't believe he would actually go through with it. I had to accept that I cannot change the past. Once I accepted that, I lightened my burden by accepting and forgiving myself. It took a lot of practice, and it's not perfect. There are hard days when shame and guilt creep back in to disturb me, but when they do, I

just return to a practice or a supporter to help release the burden, remembering some of my best qualities and focusing on those.

Sometimes, as David Kessler teaches, I add an "and" to the end of a sentence.

For example: "I am a terrible person because I wasn't kind to Glen when he called me the night before he died,"

" ... *and...* I couldn't have known it was the night before he died. I cared deeply for him, and I loved him, and I continue to love him. And, I'm a loving, caring person."

It's okay to think there is some greatness in you. It's more than okay—it's good self-care! Try repeating the practices in this book, but focus them all on forgiveness. Your journey will begin to ease.

Even with all of my therapy and mindfulness practices, it took me *four years* before I could talk out loud or write about that last conversation with Glen. That's how strong of a choke hold shame and guilt had on me. I wanted so badly to have that memory not be what actually happened, I could not speak it. Now, when I think about it, I can feel the discomfort, breathe through it, and send Glen love.

Forgiving Those Who Hurt You or Left You

This is a step on your healing journey that is best not to skip over. Once you've learned to forgive yourself (that's the harder part), you can move on to forgiving other people who might have added burdens to your journey (that's the easier part). Your backpack will feel so much lighter, and your journey will ease.

The Path They Cannot Follow and Estrangement

My hasty marriage to Glen had shaken many of my relationships, so when he died less than two years later, many of the people who had distanced themselves from me during the marriage because they disapproved didn't have any clue what to do. Maybe they felt, since they were stubbornly making their point by kicking me out of their lives that they had to stick to that stubbornness even though Glen had died. It's possible they cannot regain respect for or trust in me because even though it was so long ago, and I've grown so much, they still see me as that person I was in 2014.

Estrangement has some commonalities with death. Regardless of what I want, the relationships, as I knew them, are over. The difference is that the people are still alive and living by choice without me; the power of that rejection is devastating. And then there's the double-edged sword of hope.

Glen is dead, and even though I didn't believe it at first, eventually I fully realized and accepted he was not going to return. Our relationship is forever changed into one with him in spirit. My estrangements, however, keep a tiny bit of hope alive. There is a possibility, even if it's small, to create a positive, loving, supportive relationship with these people I have priceless history with. This hope can be incredibly destructive and retraumatizing. When I hear one of my estranged loved ones is in town and refuses to see me, it feels like another death. Grieving begins again.

Seeking Forgiveness

In Judaism, we have a tradition of asking for forgiveness and apologizing three times. If you make a sincere effort to apologize and make a situation right when your actions hurt someone, you are required to make three sincere attempts. If, after three attempts, there is no forgiveness from the person, you are no

longer responsible for the estrangement and are relieved of the burden. I tried this and am continuing to relieve myself of the burden of estrangement. Like grieving, it's an ongoing process.

Mindfulness practices have allowed me to forgive myself, and with a lot of work and practice, I have forgiven others. I do not have control over others forgiving me. Apologies, pleading for reconciliation, and promises of restitution only work if the person choosing the estrangement is willing to forgive.

There are still some relationships I yearn to repair that remain in ruins. But now I am strong enough to give those people the love and open-hearted compassion they deserve without my happiness depending on whether or not they decide to accept and forgive me. I accept that I cannot control how others think and feel. Relationships are bidirectional, and I can only open my side of the bridge. I can love them and pray for their health, happiness, and well-being. Sending them love and wishing them well feels better to me than feeling anger, betrayal, rejection, and frustration. This has all required a grieving process for these relationships, but if these loved ones come back into my life, I'll be ready to greet them with open arms and love.

How did I get here? The driving force throughout this process is *my desire to heal*. I want to feel good and enjoy my life and not hold grudges. I want a life full of love and gratitude—free of bitterness, anger, and frustration. Using the practices in this book, I came to understand I had a choice about how I feel and with whom I spend time. I don't have a choice about how other people behave; I can only choose my reaction to their behavior. I could be miserable because of the behavior of others and perpetuate those uncomfortable feelings by saying nasty things and growing my anger, or I could choose peace, compassion, and love.

Releasing guilt and blame can be so freeing and a big step toward forgiveness. Imagine it's replacing the poison with your favorite dessert—it's that sweet.

The first step to forgiveness is acceptance. We have to understand and accept that no matter how hard we wish we could, we cannot go back into the past and change what happened. We may wish we acted differently now, but we didn't, and we can't change that. But we can start there, take baby steps, and be gentle with ourselves. To achieve forgiveness, we must remember we are worthy, we are human, and we have a precious life to nurture. We deserve love and forgiveness from ourselves! Once we love and forgive ourselves, forgiveness of everyone is possible, and that is where we find true freedom.

Prayers for Them for Your Peace

Marianne Williamson, a brilliant spiritual teacher, in many of her teachings and lectures, recommends you pray for thirty days for someone you feel has hurt you. At the end of the thirty days, either your feelings toward them will shift, you will be able to release them and not care anymore, or the relationship will have shifted because of your prayers. I believe this can work with your partner. As for the people who may be adding to your suffering right now, when you feel strong enough, you can release the grip of their power to cause you suffering by practicing compassion for their suffering and letting go of expectations. Suffering is universal; we all suffer. If you can find that common ground, it can soften your heart toward those who have hurt you.

At first, the idea of forgiving someone who is behaving in a way that hurts you is nearly impossible. I resisted for a long time and instead fed my feelings of defensiveness, anger, and betrayal, which, unsurprisingly, increased my suffering. When I began to practice forgiveness and hold those who had hurt me

with compassion, the burdensome feelings of anger and betrayal lightened, my heart softened, and I suffered much less.

Forgiveness doesn't mean you agree with what the person who harmed you did. Forgiveness does not mean you approve of them or even want them back in your life. It is really about releasing yourself from the burden of carrying destructive anger with you.

Finding moments of forgiveness is like having a jet pack or a tram to help you on your journey. Forgiveness allows you to move forward by giant leaps. When I forgave all the people who made my climb steeper, who had put obstacles in my way, or who had led me off my healing path, I went from crawling along the journey to moving freely. Forgiveness is that powerful, and even more so when you practice forgiving yourself.

STAIRCASE 2

Affirmations

Affirmations are a little like meditation, and they hold a little magic. Think of them as a springboard for self-confidence and strength. If you're getting ready for a hike, you put on hiking boots, right? Affirmations are high-performance hiking boots that give your stride the lightness and power you need to make your journey easier. You may be familiar with the story *The Little Engine That Could*. His affirmation was "I think I can." He repeated this mantra to energize and reassure himself that he could get up the mountain, and he did. And you can too!

If you are about to climb the stairs to go to bed, and you are so exhausted you don't think you can make it, bring in one of my favorite affirmations: "You got this!" I talked, coached, and cheered myself on through so many difficult tasks by giving myself this simple encouragement or a "You can do this!" It helped!

Here are some more examples, and if none of these resonate with you, make up your own. Put them on a sticky note on your bathroom mirror or refrigerator. When you affirm your belief that you are going to get through this time—that you are going to be okay—your burden will lighten, the path will be illuminated, and your steps will flow.

Examples of Affirmations:

I've got this!

I am love.

I am worthy.

I release shame.

I release guilt.

I am loved.

The world is beautiful.

I am safe.

I am whole.

I will survive.

I am strong.

I can _____.

What You Say Really Matters

Words have power.

You have the power to create your new life, and it starts with your words.

Have you noticed yourself saying, "My life is over," or "My life is destroyed," or "I have nothing to live for," or some other group of heavy words? Saying these words is like adding rocks to your backpack.

Affirmations have the power to change our moods and our thoughts. Use mindfulness to stop yourself from using

disempowering words that interfere with your healing. When you're about to say something unkind or unhelpful to or about yourself, take a deep breath. Interrupt the flow of suffering and **think** kindness:

THINK*

T: Is it **true**, or is it a story that needs shifting?

H: Is it **helpful** to my healing journey?

I: Is it **impactful** in a positive way for my healing?

N: Is it **nurturing** to my healing?

K: Is it **kind** to me or my partner?

*The THINK acronym is credited to a mid-twentieth-century British pastor named Alan Redpath. It is also similar to the Three Gates of Speech offered by the Sufi poet Rumi, which are "Is it true? Is it necessary? Is it kind?" I have modified it here to make it more applicable to our healing process. If you were helping a friend go through a terrible time, would you say, "Yes, your life is over"? I am guessing not. So don't say it to yourself! Be the friend you need right now.

Even as a beginner with mindfulness and meditation practices, you can form an awareness that will allow you to notice what you say and when your words are not serving your health. I use the phrase "Let me reframe" with myself, and with clients and students, I'll ask, "How can you reframe what you just said?"

For example, when you feel as if your life is over, instead of saying, "My life is over," you can reframe it to "My life is in transition." The life you lived with your partner is over; that's true, but you will get through this difficult time and continue on to whatever your new life will hold. I know that's hard to read

or hear, but you have a life to live, when you are ready. As you journey through your grief, keep in mind that to live fully, you must grieve fully.

It's okay to say you hate this, and you can yell at your partner or the universe, God, or whomever or whatever you believe in as a higher power, to release some of that energy in motion, anytime. But when you can, also be loving toward yourself and your partner. And to support your healing, try to create mantras out of the positive, not the negative. Instead of "My life is over," say, "This too shall pass." Instead of "My life has been completely destroyed," try "I have a lot of work to do, but I can rebuild my life. And at the very least, I have my breath."

Please do not take away from this book that you are doing something wrong if you catch yourself using negative words; that would be adding pain to pain. We can all feel and say tragic things when we are grieving. That's normal and natural.

Someday, using mindfulness and careful language may help you on your healing journey. But if you do catch yourself saying something negative, it's okay! You're doing great. Thank yourself for reading this book. Deep breath!

Self-Love and Gratitude

About a year after Glen died, after I spread his ashes in the ocean, I went on a weekend retreat to one of my favorite places on earth—a rustic resort in the middle of the forest in Oregon called Breitenbush Hot Springs. No rooms were available that weekend, so I had to sign up for the retreat with the group that had all the cabins reserved. The group was called Soak in the Love, and as far as I could tell from the description, it was going to be a bit much for me to hang out with a bunch of tree-hugging hippies who like to sing and hug and pray and dance in the trees. At the time, that folksy, campy stuff sounded really dumb to me. I planned to stay in my assigned cabin and just ignore all the Soak in the Lovers. After everything I had been through that year, I felt a few days among the trees and soaking in the natural hot springs, disconnected from the outside world (Breitenbush doesn't have phone, internet, or TV), would help me heal.

The day I arrived, the retreat attendees greeted me with such warmth and compassion, I decided to go to the first night's group event. It had been too long since I had been in a group that loved and accepted me just because I was there. None of them knew anything about the last year of my life; they just looked at me like

I was a divine human, the same as them. Their acceptance of me was such a tonic for my grieving heart! I joined every meeting after that. We danced and sang songs with arm movements and hugged a lot. It reminded me of summer camp. Most of the people there had found this healing group because of deep life wounds, which, of course, resonated with me.

On the last day of the retreat, I was sitting in the meeting hall with my one hundred new best friends, and one of the teachers was answering questions from the group. Most of the people there were *A Course in Miracles* students, the minister was a teacher of this course, and this sacred text guided his answers. After he answered the third question, I noticed a theme—self-love. The solution to easing pain and ending all the self-loathing, guilt, and shame that was causing their suffering ALL ended in some version of "love yourself."

The concept surprised me, and it got me thinking: What if I was just okay with myself? What if I decided that I was just okay with all of my experiences up to this point (some of which were horrible and not at all what I would want or plan) and my behaviors (some of which were so undesirable that thinking of them filled me with shame and I struggled to accept that I had made those choices)? What if I accepted that I did all that, said all those things, felt all those feelings, and I was still okay? What if I am okay just as I am, deserving of forgiveness and love, from me? My backpack lightened so much in that single moment that my feet almost left the ground.

What if the same could be true for you?

Self-Love and Self-Compassion Practice

What if you looked at yourself right now and decided you were okay? Or even better, what if you decided you could love yourself, even with everything you've been through, even with all you've said and done leading up to this moment that you judge as bad and that you regret? What if you could forgive yourself and decide to move forward with the intention of being your best self? What if you focus on your best qualities and realize everyone is full of greatness and flaws—that we are perfect examples of the human we are meant to be? Yes, you've made mistakes. Yes, there are things you regret and wish you hadn't done, but you cannot go back and change anything. What you *can* do is apologize—to yourself and to anyone you've harmed. What if you give yourself the best opportunity to contribute to making the world a better place by accepting yourself, forgiving yourself, and now that you know better, allowing yourself to do better?

With practice, you can leave in the past the things you've done for which you feel shame, regret, or guilt. They actually *are* in the past, but we are so good at continuing to bring them forward and beating ourselves up about them.

I've heard one of my favorite stories about letting go of the past from many of my meditation teachers. As the story goes, a wise, experienced monk and a new monk in training were walking along a path that intersected a river. There was a woman on the edge of the river who was frightened to cross and needed help. The monks' vows included never touching a woman, so the young monk politely refused to help her and crossed the river safely on his own. The wise monk picked up the woman, carried her across the river, and set her down safely before the two monks continued on their journey. After several hours, the young monk stopped and turned to the older monk and said, "Master, we

made an oath not to touch a woman, yet you carried that woman across the river!" The older monk replied, "I set her down hours ago. Why are you still carrying her?"

Imagine for a moment that you leave your past behavior in the past and love and forgive the person you are right now. Then imagine that for two moments. Did you love your partner unconditionally? Do you love your kids, your pets, or anyone in your life (living or deceased) so completely that you would forgive anything they did? Turn this type of love on yourself and watch the climb flatten out and your backpack fill with light. If you can enter into self-forgiveness and self-love—if you can truly forgive and learn to love yourself—you will set yourself free. And in that freedom, you will remember and experience the love that still exists between you and your partner because love is eternal.

Gratitude

Gratitude is our emotional life support. In the same way breathing is basic life support for our physical body, gratitude is the basic life support for our emotional well-being.

There are some big ups and downs on this journey. We love the lighter times when the path flattens out, the backpack feels light, and there is no rain or snow in sight. But then that boulder rolls into the middle of the path (an estate delay, a hurtful person or activating experience, or maybe we don't even know what caused it), and we find ourselves falling back. Not into the original grief cave at the bottom of the mountain—nope, you made it out of there, and you never have to go back to those awful early times—but setbacks happen, and you may have fallen into another dark place.

What to do then?

One Dot of Gratitude

I was having a really rough day, not months but years after Glen died. I was suffering deeply that day, ruminating about painful estrangements that were still obstructing my healing. I was feeling helpless and hopeless. On top of my Glen grief at that time, I felt like I was stuck and drowning in a deep, smelly pit of quicksand over the continued estrangement of two of my primary family members—relationships I couldn't repair no matter what I did. On top of PTSD and grief, I was so focused on those losses, drowning in my suffering, that I felt I couldn't handle any more. I was in a very dark place. I started contemplating whether I had enough pills in my cabinet to end my pain permanently. If Glen could do it, so could I.

I stayed in bed, not doing any of the practices I knew would help. I just cried and suffered. I was curled up in a ball sobbing when my friend texted. We were supposed to have a phone call that morning, and I couldn't lift my head off the pillow, much less talk. I texted her, saying I just couldn't get myself up for a phone call, and gave her a small idea of how low I was feeling. When she texted me back "What are you grateful for, right now, at this moment?" I stared at the phone. I had a gratitude practice. I had a gratitude journal. I even close every yoga class I teach with a focus on gratitude. And that question made me feel like even more of a failure. I was so far from gratitude at that moment, I simply wanted to die. I threw the phone down and closed my eyes.

As time went by, and my crying was slowing, I checked my phone, and there was another text from her: "What are you grateful for, right now, at this moment?"

I took a breath, wiped my eyes and nose, and reflected. I stared at the curtains darkening my bedroom window. I wanted

149

to look around the room and try to focus on something tangible to bring me back, help me feel grounded and grateful, but it was almost completely dark in the room. Then I noticed the dot. Then I noticed more and more dots. I focused on those dots—the navy-blue polka dots in the pattern of my bedsheets. I pressed my finger onto one of the dots. I took another breath, then I picked up my phone and texted my friend. "I am grateful for my soft sheets with the blue polka dots that my sister gave me for my birthday last year."

It seems so simple, but this one moment of gratitude was lifesaving. I could almost physically feel my friend reach over and help me lift my grief backpack. It was lighter. Eventually, I got up and pulled open the curtains so my room lightened up. I drank some water. I breathed. I went to the kitchen and ate some food. Gratitude saved my life that day.

When you have a regular gratitude practice, you can not only prepare yourself for difficult times, but you can increase feelings of happiness anytime. Scientific research has proven gratitude can actually change your brain and help you live in a happier state of mind. Challenging times are easier to face if your gratitude muscle is in shape and ready to go. Just like when you train for a competition or sharpen a tool before using it, a daily gratitude practice will make it easier and more efficient to put this emotional safety net to use when you need it.

Gratitude has also been scientifically proven to improve overall health. When you are in appreciation, you cannot be in fear. Remember the bear that's chasing you? Gratitude practice is the emotional equivalent of an impenetrable bear shield.

A gratitude practice can be really easy, and the more you do it, the easier and more powerful it gets.

Gratitude Journal

Before bed, write down five things you're grateful for from your day. It may seem hard at first, but once you practice, you'll find so many things to be grateful for. It doesn't need to be anything big (a navy-blue dot on a sheet?)—it can be the air you breathe. Refocus from fretting about what you don't have and can't do to what you *do* have and *can* do. When you are in gratitude, you boost your appreciation for life and lighten your load. You can express gratitude for loved ones, the socks you're wearing, the dinner you ate, or the fact that your pen writes or your phone is charged. After you practice for a while, your list will effortlessly become endless.

When you have that gratitude muscle in shape and it becomes part of your daily life, you will have a powerful tool to protect you from despair, especially on those wet days.

Joy

Why would there be a section on joy in a book about surviving your partner's suicide? Because you are here, you are human, and you will not always feel the way you do right now. Grief, loss, trauma, guilt, sorrow, shame, and all the heavy things you are carrying right now will shift and change. Joy is our birthright, and although it may feel distant and dim right now, joy is always part of you. It may take some digging, patience, and work, but you *will* feel joy again.

When we are grieving, and something joyful happens that brings us a moment of light, it is often followed by a crash of guilt. Remember what I said earlier: All feelings are welcome—

including joy! Please, let yourself feel these moments just as deeply and clearly as you feel the pain of loss. These moments may come at odd, unexpected times, and when they do, EMBRACE THEM! You are feeding the wolf of love and strengthening your resilience!

A few days after Glen died, my helpful friend drove me to the funeral home to make arrangements, and something silly happened. Yes, at a funeral home. I had been to Jewish funeral homes, where there are only memorial cards and candles and simple coffins. Cremations, viewings, and funeral memorial takeaway gifts are not part of our tradition. When the police officer at the scene of Glen's death had asked me where I wanted the body taken after the medical examiner released it, I was too deep in shock to answer. He had suggested this funeral home, and I'd agreed.

At the funeral home, I was overwhelmed by all the urns and options for memorial items. One in particular, a bottle of barbecue sauce, labeled with the likeness of the deceased, was perched on a table in the meeting room. I completely lost it. I got hysterical, laughing and crying, looking at that bottle. Immediately, I felt guilty, but I couldn't control my laughter. At the time, I wished I had known it was okay to laugh and not shamed myself. My friend and the funeral home assistant probably wondered if I needed to be medicated or taken to the hospital, but today, I look back on that story and laugh every time I think of it. Even in a very dark place, it's possible to find joy.

The first few times you feel joy, you might reject it because you're fully encased in grieving, and it's a very difficult shift to make. You may feel you are dishonoring your partner's memory when you smile and laugh after they have died. It may seem strange to be a traumatized grieving widow and burst out laughing, but it's okay. Let yourself feel all your emotions,

especially those brief moments of joy. Forget about expectations of your behavior. You've been through a terrible, complicated loss, and however your grief manifests, it's okay!

You are still a living human, and part of being human is feeling joy. Are you going to never enjoy chocolate again? I should hope not! Eating chocolate is a great pleasure, and you are still here. You have a life to live. You are not dishonoring your partner's memory by experiencing pleasure, love, and joy. You can enjoy chocolate, or the sun on your face, and grieve your loss.

There is no shame in feeling joy, no matter what loss you have suffered.

Eventually you will have more and more moments of lightness, and you will revel in them because they will feel like a respite from your grief—a soft, shady landing to rest and refuel during your climb. Think of it as an energy boost for your healing. You'll need all the joy energy you can get to make it up this mountain you are climbing. Think of joy as a refueling station to help you get the strength you need to keep going. Take every opportunity to reconnect with the beauty and joy that are also part of our human experience. And if guilt creeps in to steal your joy, try to find reassurance that anyone who loves you, including your partner, would want you to feel joy, love, happiness, and peace.

Finding Meaning

Recently, the five stages of grieving conceived by Elisabeth Kubler-Ross (which was originally the five stages of dying) had a sixth stage officially added by David Kessler. The original five—anger, denial, bargaining, depression, and acceptance—were the standard until David lost his own son. During his grief process, he realized there was another powerful stage: finding meaning. This stage helped him on his road to recovery.

It's easy to misunderstand and even get upset by the possibility of your loved one's death having meaning, but allowing meaning to help you heal doesn't require that you find meaning in the death itself. The idea is to find the meaning in their *life* and in your own journey.

One of the basic ways to find meaning is to tell your story. Of course, we have already gone over how some people will not want to hear it; they can't hear it for whatever reasons they have. But if you tell your story to someone who can relate, you can connect with and possibly support that person, the way I'm connecting with and hopefully supporting you with this book.

It may sound like a complete stretch right now, but keep it in mind on your journey. You will come in contact with others who have suffered similar losses, and through this connection, as awful as it is, you will lessen each other's suffering because you enter into a collective suffering. The more people you can connect

with who are willing to share stories of grief and loss, the more meaning you give to your journey and theirs.

Our lives are precious, and so were the lives of those we've lost. They may no longer be here in physical form, but they live on in our hearts, and we can continue to give meaning to their lives by keeping their love alive. When we pray for our deceased loved ones in a Jewish service, we say, "They still live on earth in the acts of goodness they performed and in the hearts and minds of those who cherish their memory." The meaning of their lives can live on. Tell stories that bring you joy. Remember the unique beauty and love your partner brought into the world. And share it.

Around nine months after Glen died, I faced a difficult opportunity to practice finding meaning. Glen and I had a few really close friends while we were married. One couple, who also had married too quickly for many of their family and friends, experienced some of the same rejections and messy challenges that Glen and I had. We bonded over defending our right to love and supported each other through estrangements with our family of origin, ex-spouse challenges, and stories of how to comfort and support our children while our lives grew in love. By the time Glen died, this couple had moved out of the area, but we remained close, and because of their deep love and respect for Glen, they were a huge support to me after he died.

I noticed one day that I had missed a call from the wife. I was having a wet day, so I ignored the call because I didn't have the energy to reply. Shortly after that missed call, a visitor arrived to tell me my friend's husband had died—by suicide. I could not believe it. I refused to believe it at first. I was in shock, followed by a series of similar emotions to what I experienced when Glen died. Then I crashed into denial. This was my nervous system protecting me from overload. I couldn't take it in. I rejected the

whole thing. "Nope. No way. He couldn't have. Not right now, not so soon after Glen. Absolutely not."

"Michelle," my visitor said, "you have to call her. You're the only one who can help her. You've been through this. Call her and tell her what to do!"

"No way, I can't help her! It's too soon. I don't know what to say. I CANNOT HELP HER!" I ran crying from the room and completely rejected any conversation about the topic. For a few hours. Then I noticed a message from my friend on Facebook. She was in complete distress. I knew I needed to take a huge deep breath, ask for strength from the universe, and do what I could to support her. I had no idea what to say, but I knew she had reached out to me because she imagined I understood how she was feeling, and I could not ignore this need. It was too close, it was too much, I was still in such deep grief and PTSD, but I *did* know what she was going through. So even though I didn't think I could help, I had to at least try. I took a deep breath, picked up the phone, and stepped into service… and gave my experience meaning.

At the end of the call, she thanked me. We said a tearful goodbye and when we hung up, I cried total body sob, for hours. I did it. I supported her. And I got through it.

I didn't realize it at the time, but making that phone call was a huge boost to the resilience I would develop as I journeyed through trauma and grief. I was, or was going to be, okay. I continued to support her for the next couple of years by checking on her periodically, and whenever she reached out, I answered the phone. Each time, it got a little easier. I was able to help her in her time of need when I didn't believe I could. The strength I developed through those encounters was like taking a hundred-pound rock out of my backpack. My climb got that much easier.

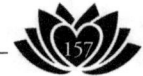

Just three months later, I got what I consider a message from the universe to write this book. Now I mentor others who have experienced the suicide loss of a partner. Mentoring and coaching others in grief helps me heal and gives meaning to my experience.

STAIRCASE 5

Faith

We grow around loss. When I was ten years old, I fell off a swing set and badly cut the front of my leg. As the wound healed, the scar spanned almost half the length of my shin. I've grown a lot since I was ten, but the scar has stayed the same size. Now its span is less than a quarter of the length of my shin and much less noticeable. It will always be there, reminding me of the pain of the wound, but also reminding me of the joyful time I had playing on that swing set. After years of growth around it, the scar is not nearly as impactful to the overall look of my leg as it once was.

The experience of losing our partner to suicide forever changes us, but we do have some input about *how* we are changed. We will never be "over" our experience, but with care and faith, we can integrate the experience into our lives in a meaningful way. Think of it as growing around the wound. The mountain you are climbing will allow you to gain strength, courage, and many skills for navigating the difficult journeys of your future. You will be able to say, "Yes, this new challenge looks tough, but when I look over my shoulder at where I've been and how far I've come, the slope doesn't appear too steep. I know I am up to the challenge— it will just be another growth opportunity."

We are all striving to grow, whether it's growing out of this terrible space we're in or beginning the basics of accepting the

place we're in. Wherever we are, we don't want to be here forever. And we won't be! When we are stuck in the grief cave, or one of the many places we will need to rest and assess, or even the spots where we trip and fall during the climb, growth is a desired byproduct of getting to the next phase. In the world of trauma-informed support, we call this resilience or post-traumatic growth. As Friedrich Nietzsche said over a hundred years ago, "That which does not kill us makes us stronger." It turns out he was right. Modern science is now providing proof that post-traumatic growth happens.

I remind you, there is no hurry. Don't add, "Oh, I should be further along than this after ___ weeks or ___ months or ___ years." Remember, no shoulding on yourself, and don't let anyone else should on you either. No one is experiencing what you are experiencing except you. Eventually, when you are ready, you will move to a place where this difficult experience will be a scar you can look at and say, "That was a difficult experience, but I have grown around it, and I am stronger for having gone through it." That may seem ridiculous at this point, which is okay. You can get there.

Building Resilience with Faith

Faith comes in many forms. Perhaps you follow a religion that supports you with faith. Maybe outside of organized religion, you have your own spiritual connection to something intangible that you believe in—God, Creator, Source, Spirit, the universe, soul, nature, divine, the Almighty, universal consciousness. During this most difficult time, connecting to and believing in something beyond the physical world can provide great comfort

and aid in healing. Again, this is your personal journey, and your relationship with the divine is also just that—yours.

Faith is the support we can cling to when the mountain gets too steep. We may not have the strength to climb, but at least we can be reassured that we will not fall. Faith is the knowing that even if we can't see beyond the curve of the path ahead, we know once we get to it, we will see the way forward to continue our journey. The ups and downs of this journey are much less scary and daunting with faith as our guide and companion. There are times when there is no other support to keep us going—no other way to continue to put one foot in front of the other. Faith reminds us we have the courage to keep going and gives us the strength to know that things will improve.

A religious or spiritual practice and a community connection that supports mourners will boost you on your journey. This is a time to contact your clergy or spiritual leader, support groups, or a focused prayer group for books or passages in sacred texts to study to bring comfort. If, however, your church is not supportive because suicide is considered a sin, this may be a time when you need to look elsewhere for support. In no way am I suggesting you leave your church. There are probably many people there who can help you at this time.

Right now, when you are in the greatest need, is not a time to be vulnerable around people who shame you or your partner. If you want to fight that battle in the future when you are stronger, great, but standing in the middle of your community in shame is like adding another thousand pounds to your backpack. Get support from the people who help you feel better. If you believe in God, love yourself as you love God and as God loves you and your partner. Doesn't that feel better than believing your partner is suffering in hell? If there is no way to know for sure, why not believe in the love-based option rather than the fear- and shame-

based option? This is a complicated, sticky, messy, tangled place. Sort it out the best you can, and if you don't know what to do, revisit your list of helpers and call one. Hang out with the people you mindfully know are helping you heal; they are here for you now. If you are going to heal, get your strength back, and get through this, you need to be with only guides, supporters, and people who lift you up. One more reminder: Don't be hard on yourself. You are doing your best. Be gentle with your mind, emotions, and body.

Whether or not you have a spiritual or religious practice, the mindfulness and meditation practices I mentioned earlier can be very helpful. Also, reading books like this one or other books about death and dying and suicide loss survival can help. Just be sure the lessons resonate with you. You can do this by checking in while you're reading—take a deep breath and feel if the book or other guide is lightening your burden or causing you to feel heavier and unsupported.

Relief and support from beyond our physical world can come from the most surprising places. Studying spiritual and religious texts about life and death and contemplating that we are eternal beings only visiting this physical world for a short time can bring great relief. Expanding my spiritual studies through the teachings of some of the great spiritual teachers, both ancient and modern, continues to help me on my healing journey. Each source of wisdom gives me a little more relief and offers something bigger than my suffering to deeply contemplate when I'm having a difficult day. Faith in something greater than myself supports me on a daily basis. As always, start small, find what feels right to you—what brings you relief—and keep trying. The most important thing is that you find something that resonates with you and helps you on your journey. When you listen to your heart and mindfully notice how you feel, you'll know which way to go.

Carefully practicing spirituality and religion, taking the wider view, zooming out to look at the bigger picture, and realizing we are part of the infinite tapestry of human history and the universe itself can drastically lighten your burden. You just have to find the right source of support—one you can connect to, one that nurtures you. It's out there; keep trying! When you bring spirituality or faith into your healing journey, the climb transforms into an opportunity for growth.

Practices to Develop Faith

1. Sit quietly and breathe slowly.
2. Try these mantras:
   - "I have faith that I will get through today."
   - "I have faith that I will be able to take one more step."
3. If that felt good, try expanding:
   - "I have faith that I will complete the _____ (task)."
   - "I have faith I will continue to breathe, eat, sleep, and move because I am in the process of recovering."
   - "I have faith that I will not always feel the way I do now."
4. If you're ready to go bigger, try this:
   - "I have faith that I will make it through this difficult time in my life, integrate this experience into my life story, and find the strength to create a life that includes this loss and also includes love and joy."

THE SUMMIT

The Journey Continues

Whew! Take a breather. You're nearing a summit!

Whether you have integrated some of the practices into your life or none of them, take a moment here to feel empowered by the fact that you opened this book at all. When you did, you took a very important step toward your healing. You decided you want to feel better.

At the summit, it's time to take another rest and assess. Get out your journal or app and write down something you've connected to in this book that you want to keep top of mind. What useful tool or practice helps you connect to your healing?

If you aren't ready to do anything other than throw this book against the wall (or at the well-meaning person who gave it to you), that's okay. You get to decide how this book will best support you. You also get to decide if it's time to rest or time to get moving.

Next Steps

You are truly an inspiration because you are here, looking for sources of support for your healing. Every word you have read and every practice you have tried is a testament to the fact that you want to heal. Deciding to heal is truly the first and most difficult step.

I need to be honest with you. The thing about grief is . . . there is no true summit. It doesn't end exactly. You don't wake up one morning and say, "I'm done grieving!"

The summit is an inconsistent place. Some days, you'll actually feel the sun on your face. You will be able to lift your chin, look back at your journey, and see the progress you've made and the strength you've built.

Some days, even the summit will feel dark and heavy. Months or even years after your loved one's death, you may encounter a pitfall and feel like you're back in your grief cave. Let me reassure you, you are not. You'll never be in that exact place again, not after how hard you've climbed. You may feel a familiar sadness or hopelessness, but you have built stamina and gathered tools on this journey that now act as a safety net. The wet days will be lighter and less frequent. And when they come, you'll know what to do. You won't add weight to your backpack by scolding yourself for "not being over it yet." On those days, you'll know to be especially kind to yourself; refer back to the self-care section of this book and take extra-good care of yourself.

There will be a day, however, with your continued commitment to your health and well-being, when you will find the grief is a smaller part of your life—that you have grown around it. More and more of your time will be spent living a fulfilling and joyful life, and less and less will be spent lost in the struggles of the grief journey. There will be a day when thoughts about your loved one will be accompanied by more love than pain.

There will be a day when feelings of compassion, gratitude, and forgiveness lift you up to much higher heights with greater power than the anger, fear, and sadness have to bring you down.

You will feel good again. You can even say that to yourself right now. Try it: "I WILL feel good again." And when you do, you can look back at your long and difficult journey and feel the meaning of your experience through your pain. The meaning *is* your strength. Hopefully, you will never again face the type of journey you are on now, but whatever you face, you will have more skills and greater strength and resilience to manage every challenge life throws your way.

The strength and the tools you developed and the practices you're doing (or might do if you haven't started yet—yes, that's okay!) to help you on your journey are yours to keep. They are part of you. You are strong and resilient. And strong, resilient people lift up our world. We need you. People are always on healing journeys—some ahead of you and some behind you. You are inspiring other journeyers to keep going. Me included.

Thank you, grief traveler.
Keep lifting yourself up. You've got this!

Answers to
Common Questions

There were so many questions I felt I couldn't answer when I began my grief journey. Most of them started with "What do I do about . . .?" or "Why . . .?" and ended with me endlessly fretting, asking everyone who would listen, and getting a lot of confused looks. People who haven't gone through this don't understand how excruciatingly difficult it is to make decisions. I mean, the first time I had to put on an outfit to go to the funeral home, it took me more than ten minutes just to choose pants. Part of this challenge to making decisions comes from the nervous system being overwhelmed by trauma. When you are under extreme stress, rational, calm thinking and decision-making are either extremely difficult or impossible. Things that may seem obvious or unimportant to anyone else may be keeping you up at night and ruminating all day.

These questions, I discovered, are very, very common.

The mindfulness practices from earlier in this book will help you make some of these difficult decisions. When you are calm, you'll have access to more of the higher-functioning and reasoning parts of your brain. You'll make more thoughtful and rational decisions and have less regret. If you take a moment to think and breathe and calm yourself before making an important decision, you're much less likely to regret your choice later. It's a really difficult time. Don't be hard on yourself if you make

a choice you regret later, but give yourself the best chance at a better outcome by slowing down and allowing your higher-thinking brain to come online.

I'm sure you're being bombarded by input and opinions from a lot of sources, some helpful and supportive, some not, but ultimately, you are the one responsible for your choices and actions going forward. I know it's new to have no partner to bounce things off of, and this is a very difficult time to grow into an independent decision-maker if you're not used to it. But you can go forward and grow through this process, starting with trusting your own choices. I'm not saying don't get help or don't ask for others' opinions on how to proceed, but also listen closely to yourself. Meditation and mindfulness practices can help you hear your inner guidance. If you think you should do something that someone encouraged you to do but doesn't feel right in your gut, then don't do it. Listen to yourself closely; mindfulness will help.

And if you need more guidance, you may find it in some of the answers below:

Q: Why does it hurt so much?

A: Your pain is a testament to how much you loved your spouse or partner. The deeper the love, the greater the pain of grief. I promise, you will not always feel the way you feel right now.

Q: Some people are being very forceful in their opinions about how I should behave, but I'm not ready to do the things they say I should be doing. What do I do?

A: Explain as clearly as you can that you are not ready to do what they think you should be doing. Here are some possible answers:

- In my current state of grief, I'm not

able to do what you're asking.

- I'm struggling with grief and doing all I can right now. Hopefully I can do what you ask soon.

- NO. (That's it. Remember, "no" is a COMPLETE SENTENCE.)

- I will think about that and get back to you.

- Grief is like an illness or an injury. If I were sick with the flu or had a broken leg, would you be expecting me to do that?

Q: Why are the people who are supposed to be my biggest supporters not helping me?

A: I covered this in detail in Part 2/Practice 5, but here's a summary. Try to keep in mind that the people closest to you are grieving too. As much as you are the primary mourner, your partner's death has a ripple effect, and all the people who knew and loved them are also suffering. When you are suffering, it's hard to support others. I know it's frustrating, but try to give them and yourself as much compassion as possible. You'll find your support. Spend more time with people who lift you up, and consider getting a therapist who is unaffected by your loss.

Q: Someone I barely know keeps calling and asking if they can come over and bring me a meal and help with things. I'm suspicious and don't feel comfortable. Should I let them help me?

A: If you're uncomfortable, you can say no or tell them to drop off something for you, maybe at a friend's house, because you aren't able to visit. It's possible this person was closer to your partner than you knew. Or maybe they have suffered a similar loss, but you two aren't close enough to have talked about it. Try

not to be suspicious, but if you aren't comfortable, simply say, "No, there's nothing I need right now."

Q: I keep fighting with my children, sister, husband's family, and I just don't have the energy to listen to what they say. I want to be a good mom, sister, daughter-in-law, but I don't know how right now. I feel so lost and incompetent. How do I handle friends and relatives?

A: This is such a tough one. I'm so sorry for these additional challenges you are facing. Keep reminding yourself that each person's grief is different. Some of your loved ones may be trying to support you but end up expressing anger instead. Your partner's death has caused a lot of stress for all of them, and while deep down they may love you and want to support you, right now they can't manage their own stress.

Repeat the mindfulness exercises and possibly the forgiveness practice. I know it's difficult, but try to hold compassion for them. Most importantly, hold compassion for yourself. You're doing your best. Keep telling yourself that.

Q: Do I bury or cremate my partner per their wishes, their family's wishes, or mine?

A: I review this in detail in Part 2, Stop 3, but I will share a bit of wisdom here for a quick answer. My mother always said, "Life is for the living." Everyone who knew your partner, even distant acquaintances, is affected by their death. People need a space to grieve. Grief needs to be witnessed. If you can help yourself and help others by following your tradition or your spouse's, that might be great. If not, do your best, and please, no matter what, do not shame yourself for making decisions here that others disagree with. You are the primary mourner, and you

need to take care of yourself and your needs. Ask yourself what feels right to you.

If you can, use the mindfulness practices from Part 1 to get in touch with yourself and really listen. You will know in your heart what to do and when.

Important Facts About Ashes:

If you do decide to spread your spouse's ashes, here are just a few things to keep in mind:

1. It doesn't have to be a one-time thing. Ashes can be spread in many places over time. If there are several precious places you think your loved one would have wanted some of their ashes, it's okay to divide them up. You can also gift some of the ashes to others who loved them if you feel right about it. Others may gain comfort from having them.

2. If someone who loved your partner wants ashes to make jewelry and you think this is the most disgusting thing you've ever heard, don't be mean to them just because they asked. Yes, this happened to me. And yes, I was very rude to the person who asked. Preserving ashes in that way grossed me out. Years later, I felt bad that I had treated her poorly and wished I could have provided some of his ashes to her. She is a jewelry maker, and this was her offering to me for Glen's memory. I couldn't appreciate it at the time, and I regret that. Just a reminder that we all grieve in our own way. We need to grieve and let others grieve.

3. Before spreading, check the wind. I've spread ashes many times. If you're going for the ocean, there's almost always a breeze coming off the waves. Hold the bag or urn close to the water and be sure the wind is at your back. You are releasing the remains of your loved one's body

to nature; you don't want them sticking to your legs.

4. When in doubt, wait. If you can't decide what to do, that means it's not time to decide. Take your time, and you will know when the time is right. If you are getting pressure from an outside source, let them know that this is your decision to make, and you will make it when you feel ready!

Q: Why doesn't anyone understand what I'm going through? This is so hard and no one gets it!

A: Your grief is your grief. No friend, therapist, family member, or other helpful person walks in your shoes. That doesn't mean they don't care. No one is going through the same thing you are. That being said, you aren't alone! Find a support group—there are many free ones online and in your local community. Look for Tender Hearts, an online grief group run by my mentor David Kessler. Find a group on Facebook, but be sure it feels supportive to be there. I joined several of these and found sometimes I would have terrible stories just popping up in my feed, so be very careful that the group you join is curated. Kristin Meekhof, author of *A Widow's Guide to Healing*, has a wonderful group for widows on Facebook.[5] It's not specific to suicide, but it is a safe, supportive place to go if you feel alone in your grief. Your grief is unique to you, but you are not alone!

Q: What do I do with their stuff?

A: I go into some detail about this in Part 2, Stop 4.

My best advice here is to take your time. If you can't stand to look at their stuff (or if you're ready to reclaim your closet space), don't get rid of anything immediately. If you have room, box it up and put it away for a while until you are further along on your journey. If you don't have room, maybe a friend has a garage or

an attic where you can keep things. As you journey through grief, your feelings about their stuff will change, so you don't want to get rid of anything too early that you may miss later.

Q: How do I find and choose a therapist who can really help?

A: Believe it or not, many people with degrees in mental health have had little or no training specifically in grief, so choose wisely. If your partner was connected to the military at all, TAPS is a great resource. If not, start with your health insurance if you have coverage for counseling and mental health. There will be a list of providers, hopefully some with training in grief. If you don't have insurance, there are foundations like The Never Alone Foundation that provide free or low-cost services. There are resources at the end of this book, Grief.com, and my website.

I detailed how to choose a therapist in Part 2, Stop 5. You can review that if you need more details.

Q: What if I need help right now and feel like I just can't go on?

A: If you are in the United States, there is an emergency line for times when you feel this way. Pick up your phone and dial 988, the Suicide and Crisis Lifeline. You are not alone.

Q: When should I take off my ring?

A: For those of you who were married, this may be a very difficult question. Glen and I were separated when he died, and during our separation, we had actually had a challenging fight about our rings. He showed up one day without his ring on, and I asked him why. We were still married, and he had said he would never take it off, so I was hurt. His response was less than kind, so I took mine off out of spite. After he died, I put on his ring and wore mine on the same finger for about a year. After I spread his ashes, I was ready to let go of that particular symbol of our

relationship. I still have the rings, and I take them out on our anniversary or other days when I miss him and wear them or hold them in my hand while I send up a prayer for his peace and mine. If it helps me feel closer to him or eases pain, then I do it.

For you, the answer is when you are ready! Not when someone else tells you to, but when you feel it is the right time. And if that time never comes, that's okay!

Q: Do I memorialize their Facebook page? Do I leave up their Instagram, Twitter, TikTok, or other digital profile?

A: This can be really tough. Glen had unfriended me on Facebook during one of our difficult times. And because I was mad at him, when he apologized and asked me to reaccept his friend request, I didn't. When he died, we weren't Facebook friends, so I couldn't access his page, including all the grief messages I needed so badly to see.

As the estate representative, I had legal rights to his digital media, and although there was a law in place in the state, both his email provider and Facebook refused to give me any access. This meant I couldn't access his computer or phone, where almost all of our photos were. While I was still working with attorneys to get access, someone told Facebook Glen had died, and they memorialized his page, which meant I had no chance to get in and re-friend myself. I was so deeply heartbroken by this. Just like with his death, I had to learn (and it took a very long time) to accept that I would have to grieve these losses as well.

If you can't access the digital media, check with your state laws to see what rights you have, or let your attorney do this. There is a new program through Stop Soldier Suicide called the Black Box Project that may be able to help you. (Check out the reference section for details.) Just take it one step at a time

and try to be patient. Keep trying and don't give up at the first no. Eventually, you may have to accept that you cannot access or change their digital world. It was another loss for me when I had to let this go. I did eventually find a hacker to get into his computer, but most of the files were inaccessible, so I never retrieved our photos, the draft he had made of his will (which would have saved me so much time and money), or any of the other things I thought I needed so badly at the time. I contacted Facebook repeatedly, and they would not budge. I learned to go on without those things. In fact, I had to use the practice of acceptance over and over again. I went through all the stages of grief again for our pictures and for his digital life.

Q: How do I tell people about what happened?

A: Like most of the answers to these questions, it will depend on how you feel. Try your best to be honest. What happened *did* happen, and keeping the truth shrouded in secrecy (where shame lives) can be hard on you and your people. If you have small children, I recommend consulting their pediatrician or a child grief specialist, or finding a children's grief book with specific age-appropriate language. Otherwise, remember, it's your story to tell. Tell as much or as little of it as you want. The questions will be endless because people have an innate curiosity about death, so try not to take their inappropriate questions personally. They really don't know better. You can't control their questions, but you do get total control over how you answer.

If you can tell your story, the more you can tell it, as long as you feel safe, the more you'll be able to move that grief energy and lighten your burden. Eventually, you will be able to help others begin their own healing journey.

Helpful Tip: Grief communities and loss specialists have shifted the way we talk about suicide to destigmatize the loss. Now we say "died by suicide" instead of "committed suicide." See how that feels when you talk about it. Committed is usually associated with a crime or a forced institutionalization. "Died by" takes the criminalization out of the term and simply allows suicide to be the way they died without the stigma.

People will ask how your spouse or partner died, especially if your partner was young. It's a basic, instinctual human curiosity that only very emotionally intelligent or grief-experienced people will be able to avoid asking. Even with all my experience and training, I still let "What did he die from?" slip in occasionally when talking with someone in grief. When someone asks, try not to let it upset you further. They aren't asking because they want to be supportive or cause you more distress. They're asking because it is natural to fear death; it's about their own fear of death. When they find out it's something that doesn't feel threatening to them, they can calm down and support you. If they are suicidal or have struggled with suicidal thoughts or actions in the past, they may have a strong reaction to your story, but it will be a swift way to realize this is not someone who can support you.

When I started telling people it was suicide, they were usually extra nice but always a little taken aback. As difficult as it is to say the words and experience the shock, horror, or pity in the eyes of the person I tell, I feel it's still best to be honest. Telling people has helped me connect with others whose lives have been touched by suicide. It allows me to feel less alone. While

I attended a meditation retreat about fifteen months after Glen died, I mentioned how I was widowed to one of the people I met. She said, "I have to introduce you to someone." She walked me over to a pair of ladies who were chatting and said, "This is my friend Michelle. Her husband died by suicide, and I thought you should meet." It turned out these other two ladies were also suicide loss survivors. One lost her son, the other her brother. We didn't spend a lot of time together and haven't kept in touch, but just that brief connection, looking deeply into these women's eyes, it was like our souls touched, and we grieved together and supported each other. So if you can, when you're ready, be open. You never know what will come back to you when you share your heart.

Q: People say things or make terrible gestures, like putting a finger to their head and pretend its a gun when they do something dumb. How do I not get triggered or activated when someone says or does something thoughtlessly that refers to suicide?

A: This is a tough one. In fact, I struggled with this a lot. Initially, I would just lose my composure and start crying because any casual reference to suicide would send me into deep grief. After doing my work in therapy and acquiring the mindfulness tools to calm myself, I would try to educate the person who made the gesture so they wouldn't do it again. The fact is that there will always be reminders that activate your trauma and grief responses, and the best you can do is learn the tools in this book so that you aren't completely thrown when you are exposed to them.

Q: All my friends have disappeared. They were around for the first weeks and months, but now they rarely return my phone calls or texts. I feel so mad and disappointed in my so-called

friends. They are supposed to be supporting me, but they have completely abandoned me!

A: Okay, that wasn't really a question, but I have heard this complaint so often in grief groups that I wanted to address it here. Like I said earlier in the book, grief (and especially suicide loss) is a really hard thing to be strong around. Your friends are still your friends, but they clearly lack the skills and strength to support you in grief. It doesn't make them bad people—just limited.

Around the time my mom died, I noticed a friend of mine had become fairly absent from my life. I cornered her in the preschool hallway one morning and asked her what was up. (I was pissed off that I had to ask her because she should have been supporting me, right?) She put her hand on my shoulder, looked me straight in the eye, and said, "Michelle, I'm sorry I haven't been around much. It just upsets me too much to see you cry."

I was so mad at her. I didn't respond, but in my head I was saying, "OH, excuse me for being sad because my mom died. I'm so sorry it's so upsetting to YOU." And a few other words may have come up as well. I was furious with her. And disappointed and hurt. If only I could have known better than to expect and demand more than people are equipped to provide. Long-term, I actually did lose that friendship permanently, but who knows why. Possibly she was so afraid of losing her own mother that she couldn't stand to be around me after I lost mine. There's no way to know what was going on for her. But that doesn't make her a bad person. Grief and loss change things. I was changed because my mother had died. Relationships change when you do. It's part of life and part of growth.

I know you need support, but right now your supporters are probably best found in grief groups and other grief-sensitive arenas. People want to go back to their lives. They want to be

okay. And they want you to be okay. If you and your friends were hiking buddies, and you broke your leg and couldn't hike with them anymore, would you expect them to sit with you until you were all healed up and then take those first few steps and then that first mile, etc., with you? They want to go hiking and you can't, so they will go hiking because they love hiking. It's not because they want to hurt you. It's because they want to enjoy hiking, and they can because, frankly, they didn't break their leg.

Your life has been affected much more than theirs by your loss. I know this might sound harsh, but I've seen so many friendships end over this, and it complicates grief even more.

It's not good for anyone. Keep in mind that ultimately, you are in this for the healing journey, and not everyone can be on it with you. Remember, they're still your friends, but they can only accompany you so far.

You can try to educate them, which is precisely why I wrote the companion's guide, *Supporting a Survivor of Spouse or Partner Suicide Loss,* that goes along with this book. You can tell them clearly what you need: "I need you to text me back when I text you to say it's my anniversary. It may seem like a long time since my partner died, but I'm really in need on this day. Can you support me?" If the answer is no, it doesn't mean they're not your friend; it just means they can't be your friend in grief. Yes, you can observe and make judgments about how lame that friend is that they can't support you, but it doesn't help you or them or your friendship to do that.

Leave them to their hiking for now and find grief support where you can. You may make some new friends through your deep connection of sharing your losses.

When you are both ready, you can have an open conversation about your experiences and decide if the friendship is something you can revive going forward. People, as challenging as they can

be, are important for our health, so don't throw anyone on the garbage heap just yet.

Q: How do I go out in public? I don't want to tell people because I don't want to bring sorrow and terror everywhere I go, but I can't always keep it together.

A: Keep in mind that you are far from the only person who is surviving suicide loss, and your friends and community want to see you thrive. (It will make them feel better.) A few months after Glen died, some close friends were having a big anniversary party. I wanted to wish them well, so I decided to go. Of course, I was very hesitant and scared. It took all my bravery (and makeup) to get myself there. When I arrived, I just hung back in the corner, not wanting to be the big dark cloud that rained on the party. The hostess came over and gave me the biggest hug. "I am so happy you are here! It's great to see you out and such a relief to know you're okay." I didn't say I was okay—I certainly was not—but I must have looked okay, and I was acting okay. The point is *she* was relieved to see me out and doing something "normal." Several other people at the party who knew my situation and knew Glen were also very kind, and I ended up feeling supported. Eventually, I knew I did the right thing by going to the party, even though I was struggling. People were happy and relieved to see me seemingly okay. And after the first few "I'm so sorry" conversations, people started treating me like just another party attendee. Honestly, it felt really good to do something a little normal for a short time.

Q: I can't stop obsessing about... What can I do?

A: There are some parts of this process that are harder than others. Those late nights ruminating about small details—the coulda shoulda woulda times—are really difficult. The mindfulness

practices I outlined earlier will help. Your therapist can help you with specifics. Do anything to help yourself build the strength to control where your thoughts go, and you can!

I had a terrible time with obsessing about a particular make and model of car. Glen died in a rental car, and that's where I found his body. After the medical examiner released the car, it was refurbished and sold. I wouldn't have thought this. I expected the car would be totaled, parted out, and crushed. A few months after he died, the rental car company sent me a $4,300 bill for repairing the damage to the car. I completely freaked out and called my insurance agent. Once I discovered that I didn't have to pay, I made the agent promise me he would take care of everything: "I do not *ever* want to see anything about this car again." They never should have sent me the bill. But I had it, and I stared at it for a long time. I didn't just file it with the hundreds of other estate-related papers. I kept staring at it. I couldn't stop thinking about the car.

And here's where I stepped off the small cliff. The VIN was on the invoice. I typed it into my computer's browser to see what would come up. There was an ad for the car, the place that was selling it, and all the details. I stepped further off the cliff and called the dealership, and when they said, "Sorry, we just sold it, but we have—" I hung up and never heard the end of that sales pitch. *The car was sold!* I couldn't get over it. I told everyone who would listen, though no one seemed quite as upset about it as I was.

Somewhere, someone was driving the car my husband died in, and they didn't even know it. Later that week, I noticed my neighbors had a new car—well, a new used car, which happened to be the same make, model, and color as THAT car. They lived three doors down from me, and every time I drove or walked by their house, I would stare at the car, wondering if it was THAT

car. I started calling this car my PTSD car because my first PTSD flashback had occurred when I saw a car like that. Every. Single. Day. I saw that car. Sometimes it distracted me so much I nearly drove off the road. I wanted to sneak over and open the door and see if the VIN matched or ask them if they had bought it at that particular used car dealership. It took a lot of therapy and some pretty advanced practices to get through this. But the point is, I did. I moved to a small condo around the corner, and I still walk by that house almost every day. Now when I see the car, I raise my hand and send it love and light. Seeing it doesn't control my behavior or feelings anymore. I'm able to breathe and release any feelings I may experience about the car or the memories associated with it. Whether or not it is the car Glen died in, it doesn't matter, because after doing that work, it's just a car that my neighbors drive.

Whatever that item is that has you spinning, see if you can use a mindfulness tool to bring love into your heart and then send it to that item. I did it with my PTSD car; you can get there too.

Q: Why?

A: This is probably the toughest question of all. If you have kids, do you remember when they were around three years old, and they went through the dreaded "WHY" phase? Some kids are so relentless that they get upset and cry if you don't give them a satisfying answer. I remember the "why" phase always came down to two responses: "Because God made it that way" or "Because I said so." This wasn't usually satisfying to the child, but at least it ended the conversation.

It's important to work hard to find your end to the conversation.

I had many, many difficult "whys" I eventually made it through.

Why couldn't I find a will? Why did he empty our bank account before he died? Why did he take his life when he has three beautiful children and three beautiful step-children?

The easiest and most difficult way to get through the "why" phase is to let them go. Back to the practice of acceptance. Most of these "whys" are unanswerable, and if you can't answer the unanswerable question, you will never find peace until you can let it go. Answer your question with this question: What helps you?

Mindfulness can help you get control of that endless ruminating and more easily shift to figuring out what helps you. Does finding out the answer to that "why" change anything? Does it change the past or your current situation? Most likely not.

One idea that might help if there is no way to get the actual answer to one of your "whys" is writing it out. As I mentioned earlier, writing is a way to process emotions by giving them a way to move through your mind.

Write down the question and all the possible answers. Pray or meditate silently and see if one of the answers feels like the best one. Even if you don't get an answer, this process will help you move some of the feelings that are spinning around in your head and give you some relief.

Q: Why are my kids acting like they're fine? Or why are my kids acting so horribly? Or why are my kids . . .?

A: Kids, depending on their age, will grieve in unexpected ways. They may not cry at all and act fine and want to be with their friends, or they may just want to stay in bed. Keep reassuring them that you love them and you are there for them. Have as honest, open, and age-appropriate conversations with them as you feel is possible. Taking care of yourself the best you can is the best way to demonstrate healthy grieving. It's so difficult because you want to take away their pain, but as I mentioned

earlier, you cannot grieve for them. This is a process they need to go through and, eventually, with your love and support, grow through. There are many helpful books and videos about children and grieving. Search for one that matches your children's ages and resonates with you. Ask your helpers to do this research if it's too much for you.

Q: When do I...?

A: You have probably figured out the answer to this one by now: Exactly when you feel you are ready!

Talking with other spouse/partner suicide loss survivors, I have a consensus about a few things I can share with you:

If you can, avoid making any major decisions for at least a year. This includes relocating, changing jobs, or making major purchases. If you need to do anything like this, ask a trusted friend or therapist for reassurance that you are making the best decision for your healing journey. The practices I've shared in this book will help you be in your clearest state, but it's still very difficult to make wise choices while you're deep in your grief cave and sometimes even while you're on your climb.

If you don't have to make the change or big decision now, wait.

Resources and References

Here are some resources you may find helpful as you continue your journey as well as specific references to some of the resources I mentioned in the book.

Communities with Information and Support

Grief.com offers information, courses, and a community to support those in grief.

TAPS (Tragedy Assistance Program for Survivors) is a great resource if your spouse or partner served in any capacity. www.taps.org

Stop Soldier Suicide and the Black Box Project helps suicide loss survivors to access information on the devices of veterans while working to identify trends that will increase prevention efforts. www.stopsoldiersuicide.org/blackboxproject

Soaring Spirits International is an inclusive community with support for anyone who has lost a partner. They also offer help to supporters of those who have lost a partner. www.soaringspirits.org

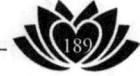

Hotline

988 Suicide and Crisis Lifeline in the USA

Canada—Talk Suicide: 1.833.456.4566

UK—Samaritans: 116 123

South Africa Suicide Crisis Line: 0800.567.567

Blog/Article

Mayo Clinic Staff. "Suicide Grief," *Healthy Lifestyle*. August 5, 2022. https://www.mayoclinic.org/healthy-lifestyle/end-of-life/in-depth/suicide/art-20044900

Books about Partner Loss

Ashton, Jennifer. 2019. *Life After Suicide: Finding Courage, Comfort & Community after Unthinkable Loss*. New York: HarperCollins.

Meekhof, Kristin, and James Windell. 2015. *A Widow's Guide to Healing: Gentle Support and Advice for the First 5 Years*. Naperville, IL: Sourcebooks.

Rasmussen, Christina. 2013. *Second Firsts: Live, Laugh, and Love Again*. Carlsbad, CA: Hay House.

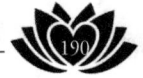

Books about Grief and Healing

Hay, Louise, and David Kessler. 2014. *You Can Heal Your Heart: Finding Peace After a Breakup, Divorce, or Death*. Carlsbad, CA: Hay House,

Kessler, David. 2019. *Finding Meaning: The Sixth Stage of Grief*, p. 228. New York: Simon & Schuster.

References

1. David Kessler. Releasing the Guilt of Grief. July 19, 2022. https://grief.com/podcast/releasing-the-guilt-of-grief/

2. Brown, Brené. 2018. *Dare to Lead.* New York. Random House.

3. Zach Bush, MD. "4 Minute Workout," September 5, 2017. https://youtu.be/PwJCJToQmps

4. https://griefyoga.com/

5. https://www.facebook.com/KristinMeekhof

About
Michelle Ann Collins

As the founder of Inhabit Joy, Michelle Ann Collins partners with individuals who have suffered grief, injury, or other types of loss as they recover, reclaim their wholeness, and build resilience for life's inevitable challenges. After a series of losses, including the death of her mother, her husband's suicide, and continued estrangements from primary family members, Michelle combined the tools she had collected as a yoga therapist and wellness coach and studies in positive psychology, neuroscience, meditation and mindfulness, and spirituality to turn post-traumatic stress disorder into post-traumatic growth and resilience. With the addition of a certification in grief education and several bestselling books in which she shares her story, Michelle is helping others transform from barely surviving to joyful thriving.

Deeply connected with the healing powers of nature, Michelle spends her leisure time hiking among the trees or paddling on the rivers near her home in Portland, Oregon.

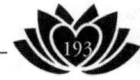

A Special Invitation

Your healing journey has begun. What's your next step? Would you like more support from someone who understands?

Take the Next Step in Mindful Healing

At Inhabit Joy, I help individuals who have suffered grief, injury, and loss as they recover, reclaim their wholeness, and build resilience for life's inevitable challenges.

Private and Group Yoga Sessions
Meditation and Support Groups
Private and Group Coaching Programs

If you're not sure which next step will be most helpful on your journey, book a free consultation at

www.InhabitJoy.com.